PHYSICAL THERAPY MANAGEMENT of ARTHRITIS

Edited by

Barbara F. Banwell, M.A., P.T.

Lecturer
Physical Therapy Program
The University of Michigan—Flint
School of Health Sciences
Flint, Michigan

Victoria Gall, M.Ed., P.T.

Rehabilitation Coordinator
Orthopedics and Rheumatology
Rehabilitation Services
Brigham and Women's Hospital
Boston, Massachusetts

CHURCHILL LIVINGSTONE
NEW YORK, EDINBURGH, LONDON, MELBOURNE
1988

Library of Congress Cataloging-in-Publication Data

Physical therapy management of arthritis.

  (Clinics in physical therapy ; v. 16)
  Includes bibliographies and index.
  1. Arthritics—Rehabilitation.   2. Physical therapy.
I. Banwell, Barbara F.   II. Gall, Victoria.   III. Series.
[DNLM: 1. Arthritis—rehabilitation.   2. Physical
therapy.   W1 CL831CN v.16 / WE 344 P578]
RC933.P47   1988   616.7'22062   87-24978
ISBN 0-443-08438-6

© Churchill Livingstone Inc.   1988

Distributed in the United Kingdom by Churchill Livingstone,
Robert Stevenson House, 1-3 Baxter's Place, Leith Walk,
Edinburgh EH1 3AF, and by associated companies, branches,
and representatives throughout the world.

Acquisitions Editor: *Kim Loretucci*
Copy Editor: *Ann Ruzycka*
Production Designer: *Jill Little*
Production Supervisor: *Jane Grochowski*

Printed in the United States of America

First published in 1988

Contributors

Barbara F. Banwell, M.A., P.T.
Lecturer, Physical Therapy Program, The University of Michigan—Flint, School of Health Sciences, Flint, Michigan

Lenora W. Barnes, P.T.
Staff Therapist, Physical Therapy Department, C. S. Mott Children's Hospital, Ann Arbor, Michigan

Eric P. Gall, M.D.
Professor and Chief, Section of Rheumatology, Department of Internal Medicine, and Professor, Departments of Surgery (Orthopedics) and Family and Community Medicine, University of Arizona College of Medicine, Tucson, Arizona

Victoria Gall, M.Ed., P.T.
Rehabilitation Coordinator, Orthopedics and Rheumatology, Rehabilitation Services, Brigham and Women's Hospital, Boston, Massachusetts

Kathleen Haralson, P.T.
Clinical Specialist, Division of Rheumatology, Department of Internal Medicine, Washington University School of Medicine, St. Louis, Missouri

Phyllis Levine, P.T.
Chicagoland Orthopedic Rehabilitation Services, Ltd., Palos Heights, Illinois

Peggy T. McKnight, O.T.R.
Consultant, Department of Occupational Therapy, St. Margaret Memorial Hospital, Pittsburgh, Pennsylvania

Carolee Moncur, Ph.D., P.T.
Associate Professor, Division of Physical Therapy, and Consultant, Division of Rheumatology, Department of Internal Medicine, University of Utah School of Medicine, Salt Lake City, Utah

Linda K. Schroeder, P.T.
Physical Therapy Division, University of Michigan Hospitals, Ann Arbor, Michigan

Preface

Arthritis may well be the diagnosis most commonly encountered by physical therapists. As a primary or secondary condition, it is the source of countless patient problems and disabilities. Arthritis, of course, is not a single disease but a category of diseases that includes over 100 separate entities. Physical agents and exercises have been used to relieve problems related to arthritis since early times and in all parts of the world. Physical therapy has long been regarded as a basic component of arthritis treatment programs and the physical therapist an integral member of the treatment team.

Interestingly, arthritis has not received a great deal of attention from the professional community of physical therapists until the past few years. Previously very little research was done in the area, few arthritis-related papers were presented at scientific meetings, and the basic treatment regimens remained unchanged and unchallenged. Many physical therapists viewed the treatment of people with arthritis as relatively basic and without challenge. Treatment programs consisting of heat, range of motion, isometric exercises, and rest were the rule. However, this lack of excitement for arthritis treatment changed in the 1970s with the establishment of Multipurpose Arthritis Centers by the National Institutes of Health. These centers emphasized comprehensive care and sought innovative and effective treatments from many professional disciplines, including physical therapy. Patient education and community programs were developed and evaluated. Research funds were available for the investigation of new and old treatment activities. An attitude of inquiry was established and physical therapy for arthritis was seen in a new light. Physical therapists involved with Multipurpose Arthritis Centers (MACs) learned research methodology and were able to establish liaisons with other investigators to facilitate their research activities. Parallel to the development of the MACs was the growth of the Arthritis Health Professions Association, the professional organization of the Arthritis Foundation. This organization provides a means for health professionals interested in arthritis to interact and exchange ideas and to influence policy.

The results of the past ten years of activity in rheumatology have been extraordinary. More is now understood about the pathophysiology of rheumatic disease, the mechanisms of pharmaceutical actions, and the efficacy of treatment. Physical therapy treatment activities have also changed. New philosophies about exercise, in particular, have emerged, as well as an improved understanding and application of physical agents.

This book is intended for all physical therapists at every level of proficiency. Because arthritis is a diagnosis encountered so often, therapists should be as knowledgeable as possible about its treatment. The contributors to this book view the treatment of arthritis as an exciting and challenging area of physical therapy practice. While many of the treatment activities are relatively basic, decision-making for treatment is essential and such decisions must be based on knowledge and experience. We hope that some of that knowledge can be gained from this book. Although most forms of arthritis cannot be cured at this time, the potential for effective management is significant, and physical therapy is essential to that management.

Barbara F. Banwell, M.A., P.T.
Victoria Gall, M.Ed., P.T.

Contents

1 | Pathophysiology of Rheumatic Disease

Eric P. Gall

The list of rheumatic diseases is long and the pathogenesis of many complicated. Specialists in rheumatic diseases are called upon to see over 100 different ailments. There are several different unifying concepts to these lists that help to cement the relationships. In one case many of these illnesses afflict the musculoskeletal system as the sole or one of several organ systems. A number of diseases are immune, particularly autoimmune or immune complex in origin. The variety of diseases has been codified by a committee of the American Rheumatism Association (Table 1-1).[1]

Major advances in understanding the pathogenesis of these illnesses has occurred in the last several decades. The recognition of these accomplishments was made at the 50th Anniversary of the American Rheumatism Association in a "Landmark Discoveries" symposium in 1984.[2]

It has been my observation that success with "definitive" treatment and or cure of diseases is directly related to the understanding of the pathogenesis of that disease. For instance, while we know much about the cause of rheumatoid arthritis, our knowledge is still in flux. The disease was not clearly defined until 1958 and there has been much argument about the classification since then.[3] The disease was not even well described until Beauvais did so in his doctoral thesis in 1800.[4] We now can control the disease in many instances but our therapy continues to evolve and definitive treatment indeed is in the future.[5] On the other hand, gout has been well understood for many years. Van Leuwenhoke described the sodium urate crystals in the tophus many years ago. The uric acid metabolic pathways and enzymatic control mechanisms as well as the renal handling of uric acid was fully described during the 1950s and 1960s. As a logical sequel to understanding the cause of the disease, this lead to the development of drugs capable of fully preventing this disorder. If the

1

Table 1-1. Classification of the Rheumatic Diseases

I. Diffuse connective tissue diseases
  A. Rheumatoid arthritis
  B. Juvenile arthritis
    1. Systemic onset
    2. Polyarticular onset
    3. Oligarticular onset
  C. Systemic lupus erythematosus
  D. Progressive systemic sclerosis
  E. Polymyositis/dermatomyositis
  F. Necrotizing vasculitis and other vasculopathies
    1. Polyarteritis nodosa group (includes hepatitis B, associated arteritis, and Churg-Strauss allergic granulomatosis)
    2. Hypersensitivity vasculitis (includes Schonlein-Henoch purpura and others)
    3. Wegener's granulomatosis
    4. Giant cell arteritis
      a. Temporal arteritis
      b. Takayasu's arteritis
    5. Mucocutaneous lymph node syndrome (Kawasaki's disease)
    6. Behcet's disease
  G. Sjögren's syndrome
  H. Overlap syndromes (includes mixed connective tissue disease)
  I. Others (includes polymyalgia rheumatica, panniculitis (Webber-Christian disease), erythema nodosum, relapsing polychondritis and others)

II. Arthritis associated with spondylitis
  A. Ankylosing spondylitis
  B. Reiter's syndrome
  C. Psoriatic arthritis
  D. Arthritis associated with chronic inflammatory bowel disease

III. Degenerative joint disease (osteoarthritis, osteoarthrosis)
  A. Primary (includes erosive osteoarthritis)
  B. Secondary

IV. Arthritis, tenosynovitis, and bursitis associated with infectious agents
  A. Direct
    1. Bacterial
      a. Gram-positive cocci (staphylococcus and others)
      b. Gram-negative cocci (gonococcus and others)
      c. Gram-positive rods
      d. Mycobacteria
      e. Treponemes
      f. Others
    2. Viral
    3. Fungal
    4. Parasitic
    5. Unknown, suspected (Whipple's disease)
  B. Indirect (reactive)
    1. Bacterial (includes acute rheumatic fever, intestinal bypass, postdysenteric-shigella, yersinia, and others)
    2. Viral (hepatitis B)

V. Metabolic and endocrine diseases associated with rheumatic states
  A. Crystal-induced conditions
    1. Monosodium urate (gout)
    2. Calcium pyrophosphate dihydrate (pseudogout, chondrocalcinosis)
    3. Hydroxyapatite

(Continued)

Table 1-1. Classification of the Rheumatic Diseases (*continued*)

   B. Biochemical abnormalities
      1. Amyloidosis
      2. Vitamin C deficiency (scurvy)
      3. Specific enzyme deficiency states (including Fabry's, Farber's, alkaptonuria, Lesch-Nyhan and others)
      4. Hyperlipidemias (types II, IIa, IV)
      5. Mucopolysaccharides
      6. Hemoglobinopathies (sickle cell disease and others)
      7. True connective tissue disorders (Ehlers-Danlos, Marfan's, pseudoxanthoma elasticum, and others)
      8. Others
   C. Endocrine diseases
      1. Diabetes mellitus
      2. Acromegaly
      3. Hyperparathyroidism
      4. Thyroid disease (hyperthyroidism, hypothyroidism)
   D. Immunodeficiency diseases
   E. Other hereditary disorders
      1. Arthrogryposis multiplex congenita
      2. Hypermobility syndromes
      3. Myositis ossificans progressiva

VI. Neoplasms
   A. Primary (e.g., synovioma, synoviosaracoma)
   B. Metastatic

VII. Neuropathic disorders
   A. Charcot joints
   B. Compression neuropathies
      1. Peripheral entrapment (carpal tunnel syndrome and others)
      2. Radiculopathy
      3. Spinal stenosis
   C. Reflex sympathetic dystrophy syndrome (RSDS)
   D. Others

VIII. Bone and cartilage disorders associated with articular manifestations
   A. Osteoporosis
      1. Generalized
      2. Localized (regional)
   B. Osteomalacia
   C. Hypertrophic osteoarthropathy
   D. Diffuse idiopathic skeletal hyperostosis (DISH) (includes ankylosing vertebral hyperostosis-Forrestier's disease)

IX. Nonarticular rheumatism
   A. Myofascial pain syndromes
      1. Generalized (fibrositis, fibromyalgia)
      2. Regional
   B. Low back pain and intervertebral disc disorders
   C. Tendinitis (tenosynovitis) and/or bursitis
      1. Subacromial/subdeltoid bursitis
      2. Bicipital tendinitis, tenosynovitis
      3. Olecranon bursitis
      4. Epicondylitis, medial or lateral humeral
      5. DeQuervain's tenosynovitis
      6. Adhesive capsulitis of the shoulder (frozen shoulder)
      7. Trigger finger
   D. Ganglion cysts
   E. Fascitis
   F. Chronic ligament and muscle strain

(Continued)

Table 1-1. Classification of the Rheumatic Diseases (*continued*)

G. Vasomotor disorders
   1. Erythromelalgia
   2. Raynaud's disease or phenomenon
H. Miscellaneous pain syndromes (includes weather sensitivity, psychogenic rheumatism)

X. Miscellaneous disorders
  A. Disorders frequently associated with arthritis
    1. Trauma (the result of direct trauma)
    2. Lyme arthritis
    3. Pancreatic disease
    4. Sarcoidosis
    5. Palindromic rheumatism
    6. Intermittent hydrarthrosis
    7. Villonodular synovitis
    8. Hemophilia
  B. Other conditions
    1. Internal derangement of joints (includes chondromalacia patella, loose bodies)
    2. Familial Mediterranean fever
    3. Eosinophilic fasciitis
    4. Chronic active hepatitis
    5. Other drug-induced rheumatic syndromes

(Rodnan GP, Schumacher HR: Primer on Rheumatic Diseases. 8th ed. The Arthritis Foundation, Atlanta 1983.)

information is properly applied to treatment, clinical gouty arthritis can be a disease of historical interest only.

It would be impossible to discuss the pathophysiology of all the rheumatic diseases in complete detail. For this reason we will utilize a few representative examples and discuss what is known of their causes as they relate to the treatment. We will cover rheumatoid arthritis and osteoarthritis in more detail and present some information on gout, ankylosing spondylitis, (and related axial arthropathies), and pyogenic septic arthritis. References will be given to cover more comprehensive detail of these and other diseases.

RHEUMATOID ARTHRITIS

As alluded to earlier regarding the pathogenesis of rheumatoid arthritis (RA), much is known; much is yet to be learned. In the years gone by, RA was considered to be caused by a bacterial agent. Cecil reported agglutination of the streptococcus by serum of patients with RA, suggesting this organism to be etiologic.[6] This has been subsequently disproved by showing the agglutination was a nonspecific antibody to the antistreptococcal gamma globulin coating the bacteria. In 1948, the discovery of the rheumatoid factor by Rose and Waller provided the first clue to pathogenesis of rheumatoid arthritis.[7] The factor is an antibody to human IgG, an autoantibody, and is measured in the routine laboratory as will be noted later. Although other rheumatoid factors are present (IgG, and IgA-anti IgG) the actual part they play in causing the disease is not known. In 1965 Hollander suggested that rheumatoid factor and gamma globulin combined to form immune complexes in the joint and thus

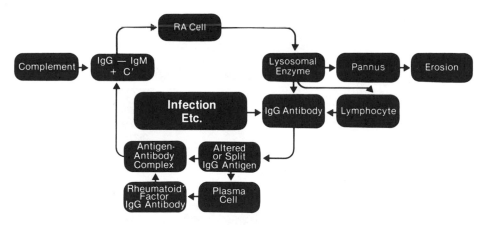

Fig. 1-1. Hollander model of pathogenesis of rheumatoid arthritis. (Modified from Hollander JL, McCarty DJ, Astorga G, Rawson AJ: Studies on the pathogenesis of rheumatoid joint inflammation. 1. The RA cell and a working hypothesis. Ann Int Med 62:271, 1965.)

excite an inflammatory response[8] (Fig. 1-1). Since that time, the story has become far more complex as depicted by a complicated arborization, "Rheumatoid Roots," which shows some of the more recent information (Fig. 1-2). Indeed not all mechanisms may be operative at the same time. Some may affect others by either positive or negative feedback and control. All have important therapeutic considerations, which in some cases may require more than one medication or other interventions for optimal control. Important players in this scenario of the pathogenesis include initiating factors, genetic predisposition, the cellular and humoral immune system, complement, the neutrophil, macrophage, synovial cell and chondrocyte, cellular enzymes, interleukines, kinins, connective tissue activating peptides, tissues such as cartilage, synovium, and bone, the arachidonic acid system, and physical and psychological factors. Obviously a thorough discussion of all of these would involve an entire book in and of itself. We can only touch the surface by identifying some of these factors in more detail.

If one were able to tackle the initiating factors and eliminate them, there would be little need of understanding the rest. Prevention would preclude the need for treatment. The problem is that the potential initiating factors are probably multiple and ubiquitous, thus difficult to prevent. For many years the search for a viral cause for RA has continued. The problem that occurred is most studies are done on established disease. By this time a virus may have triggered a sequence of events but may no longer be present. Likewise viral genetic material may be incorporated into cells and antigenic viral coating, etc. and no longer may be detectable. Direct viral culture and co-culture techniques have been unsuccessful in finding etiologic agents. Prospective studies in early synovitis before the diagnosis is known will be helpful and are in progress in this and other institutions. These could identify organisms before they are degraded and lost.

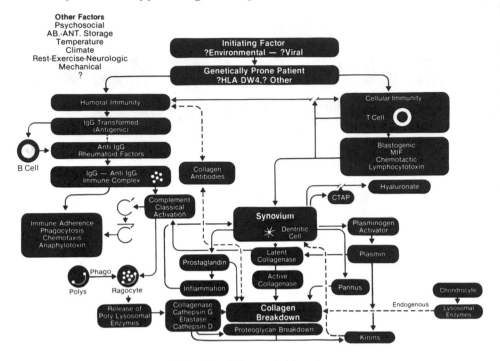

Fig. 1-2.   Rheumatoid roots.

Viral–like particles have been found in the synovium of patients with RA but are not proven to be virus. An antigen related to the Epstein–Barr virus (RANA) has been found to react with serum of patients with rheumatoid arthritis.[9] Epstein–Barr virus (EBV) is known to be able to cause lymphocyte proliferation and B-cell activation. Others have found that this antibody is not specific for RA. Other studies have not yet implicated the virus as etiologic in RA but there is continued intrigue with this possibility.

Perhaps various viruses are one of several possible triggers to the disease. Other studies have implicated the possibility that mycoplasma and bacterial cell walls might begin an immune response that will eventually result in rheumatoid disease.

The genetic factor of susceptibility to rheumatoid arthritis is better substantiated. The D-related cell surface alloantibody of the HLA system has been typed. The HLA-DR4 antibody is present in over 70 percent of patients with RA but in only 28 percent of controls.[10] This is less spectacular than the linkage of HLA-B27 to spondylitis but suggests, that a linked gene causes patients to be susceptible to RA. This may be added to the fact that females manifest rheumatoid arthritis two to four times more commonly than males and that certain populations have a very high incidence of the illness.

Immunologic mechanisms for the development and perpetuation of rheumatoid arthritis are very important. Lymphocytes are involved—both the humoral (B cell, or plasma cell),[8] and the cellular (T cell) systems are involved.

The B cell is responsible for antibody formation. The best known antibody involved with rheumatoid arthritis is the so–called "rheumatoid factor." This antibody is an antibody to human gamma globulin that has become antigenic possibly because of the alteration of its tertiary structure by some of the initiating mechanisms previously discussed.

The presence of rheumatoid factors is measured in the routine laboratory by agglutination of latex particles covered by IgG (thus altering the conformation) or by sheep red blood cells covered with an IgG antibody to them. These laboratory methods only measure IgM rheumatoid factors (anti-IgG) but not IgG and IgA factors, which may be present along with or exclusive of the IgM factor. Thus some patients with actual rheumatoid factors will be missed by the commonly available methodology. This may account for the approximately 20 percent of patients with RA who are "seronegative."

To interpret the presence of rheumatoid factor one must know the titer, being significant only at 1:160 or greater with the latex test and 1:32 or greater with the sheep cell agglutination test (SCAT). Despite this, the sensitivity of the latex reaction is 75 to 80 percent and the specificity about 75 percent. The test is more likely to be positive in severe progressive disease particularly with systemic manifestations such as rheumatoid nodules. Sjögren's syndrome, Felty's syndrome, and leg ulcers. The older the patient is, the more likely that patient is to test positive for a significant titer of rheumatoid factor. Patients without rheumatoid arthritis but who have chronic infections (chronic bronchitis, subacute bacterial endocarditis) chronic fibrotic disease (pulmonary fibrosis, cirrhosis), and a variety of other conditions may also have false-positive rheumatoid factors in significant titers.

The SCAT test is far more specific than the latex test. Ninety percent of the patients with a positive test have rheumatoid arthritis. This specificity is only gained with a loss of sensitivity. Only 50 percent of RA patients have a positive SCAT rheumatoid factor test.

The rheumatoid factor is thought to participate in the pathogenesis of RA by forming an immune complex with human gamma globulin. This complex then activates the complement system and complement in turn causes neutrophils to be attracted to the immune complex (chemotaxis), particularly in the joint. The neutrophils then phagocytize the immune complex and in the process of doing so release toxic enzymes into the surrounding milieux. These proteases, collagenases, and cathepsins cause the synovium to proliferate and become inflamed. They also cause cartilage and bony destruction by invasion called pannus. Simultaneously, the immune complexes are stored in articular cartilage and synovium, causing chronicity of the inflammatory response.

Drugs that might inhibit the rheumatoid factor production and immune complex formation are primarily the "remittive agents" such as gold, penicillamine, and cytotoxic agents. Gold also inhibits complement activation. The anti-inflammatory drugs (aspirin and the newer nonsteroidal anti-inflammatory drugs—"NSAIDs") inhibit the activation of neutrophils. Some physical modalities (heat, active exercise) may aggravate the inflammatory response in some instances and patients must be monitored to make sure this does not occur.

The cellular immune response is also active in rheumatoid arthritis. How they are activated is not known but T cells become "turned on," release lymphokines (humoral inflammatory substances), and depending on which subset is involved may aggravate or ameliorate the humoral immune response. Helper (inducer) T cells cluster around macrophages in the synovium. The macrophage is a phagocytic cell that processes antigen for presentation to the T cells and the activated T helper cells induce B cells to form immunoglobulin (e.g., rheumatoid factors). Once again the remittive agents are most likely to aid in controlling the cellular immune response in rheumatoid arthritis.

While the lymphocyte and neutrophil are obviously important in rheumatoid arthritis, other cells are involved. Macrophages are activated by whatever the initiating process is for RA and they produce interleukin 1, angiogenesis factors (causing proliferation of capillaries), and toxic enzymes, all of which cause further inflammation and destruction. For unknown reasons the chondrocyte in the cartilage also begins to secrete collagenase which destroys the collagen it has just produced, a so called suicide phenomenon. Other cells such as mast cells proliferate in the joint tissues. The net result of all these inflammatory cells is the release of further inflammatory mediators including kinins, leukotrienes, prostaglandins, and free oxygen radicals. These then add to the vicious cycle of joint destruction and further cellular proliferation.

What has been illustrated in this lengthy discussion of active mechanisms in the pathogenesis of RA is a multifactorial etiology with some unanswered questions. The intricate interplay of pathways makes one realize that interference with one mechanism may, indeed, increase another. One also realizes that therapy (pharmacologic, modalities, and others) may be complex requiring several simultaneous interventions. Close monitoring for the activity status of the disease is requisite. Because of the complex interactions, therapy that is efficacious in some instances is harmful in others. Only the health professional in cooperation with the patient can determine this through careful monitoring. New research for new treatment methods is mandatory also. This is particularly true in the nonpharmacologic modalities of care. The question is raised as to whether they are helpful, harmful, and in what instances they should be used. This is particularly important in these days of more difficult third party payments for arthritis care.

DEGENERATIVE JOINT DISEASE, OSTEOARTHRITIS

While less complicated, degenerative joint disease (osteoarthritis, DJD) also has less known about its pathogenesis than rheumatoid arthritis. A few years ago there was a move in the United States to use the British terminology and call this most common type of arthritis in man osteoarth*rosis* rather than -*itis* (the latter connoting inflammation). The reason for this is if one examines the synovium and synovial fluid of these patients little inflammatory infiltrate is seen. Most health professionals in dealing with these patients noted that heat, swelling, fluid, and some of the other cardinal signs of inflammation were present despite the benign nature of the tissues. Now we realize that crystal deposition, both hydroxyapetite and calcium pyrophosphate and perhaps others, may excite some inflammation and lead to mild to moderate inflammation in some people. Thus the terminology, "osteoarthritis" may indeed be appropriate. In addition, friction and other physical forces cause inflammatory changes. Nonetheless, the synovial fluid seldom contains more than 1000 to 2000 WBCs/mm³ and is classified as noninflammatory. The reason for this supposed contradiction is unclear.

Another misconception concerning this disease was that it was primarily a disease of the elderly and only caused by "wear and tear." Recent information suggests that there is a genetic predisposition to the disease, a number of causative metabolic abnormalities, and further worsening by structural, physical, and anatomic incongruities.

Clinically, the disease tends to involve fewer joints than rheumatoid arthritis. It is also more asymmetric than RA. Not only will it involve one side of the body and not the contralateral side in many cases, but it is also asymmetric within the joint, involving either the medial or lateral portion of the knee, but not the other. While rheumatoid arthritis is a bone wasting (osteopenic) disease, osteoarthritis is a bone forming disease. Radiographically, it is characterized by asymmetric joint space narrowing due to cartilage loss, with reactive new bone formation where bone rubs on bone. It is as if the body is attempting to repair the damage to the cartilage by buttressing the adjacent bare bone. Indeed, in an attempt to widen the articular surface and thus better distribute the load caused by the disease, bony spurs (osteophytes) are formed at the edge of the bone. These are not usually seen with inflammatory arthritis. The exception to this is when an inflammatory arthritis burns out and goes into remission. The joints that are then left permanently damaged may develop secondary osteoarthritis. Subchondral cysts are seen in osteoarthritis and while they also may be found in RA, marginal erosions of bone are more likely to be seen in the latter. These cysts may collapse under the pressure of weight bearing causing severe articular destruction. Clinical swelling of the joints is often hard and boney due to the osteophytes, although fluid is also present particularly in weight bearing joints. It is rare in DJD to feel "mushy" or "doughy" proliferative synovium about the joint.

The study of the pathogenesis of DJD leads one to the careful analysis of the synthetic biochemistry of cartilage and bone. Only recently has much emphasis been put into research in this area.

Cartilage serves as a weight–bearing covering and cushion at the end of bone. It is avascular and receives its nourishment by acting as a sponge, thus soaking up synovial fluid. It eliminates its metabolic waste products by compressing the sponge pushing the fluid back out of the tissue. Thus exercise movement and force upon the joint is requisite for maintenance of cartilage. The cells (chondrocytes) make up only about 5 percent of the total cartilage mass. These cells synthesize and secrete the bulk of the rest of the cartilage, the matrix material (proteoglycans, 50 percent of the dry weight), and the strong skeletal material, collagen (10 percent). Water is present in substantial amounts.

Glycosaminoglycans (GAG, or mucopolysacharrades) include keratin and chondroitin SO_4, which vary in quantity with the place they occur in the cartilage, the patients age, and the amount of damage occuring. Chondroitin SO_4 increases secondary to stress in weight-bearing regions of the joint. Experimental changes in joint supporting structures cause marked alterations in glycosaminoglycan (GAG) distribution. Trauma to the joint initially causes an increase in GAG synthesis. These glycosaminoglycans are bound to proteins to form proteoglycans. This structure resembles a centipede with the GAG sticking out from a hyaluronic acid core. Water is attracted to be interspersed within the structures. This gives cartilage much of its resiliant character.

Scattered throughout the proteoglycan matrix are collagen strands that give cartilage its strength. Depending on the depth, they are either parallel to the surface (superficial) or perpendicular (deeper layers). Type II collagen is the predominate type in cartilage and is chemically unique. In disease, the types of cartilage may change to other less desirable types.

The chondrocyte produces proteoglycans, link proteins, collagen, and hyaluronic acid, and also regulates their degradation with proteolytic enzymes. The synthesis and catabolism are strongly influenced by the extracellular mileau. Synovial macrophages secrete a material called catabolin (interleukin I), which causes chondrocytes to secrete collagenase and proteases, which in turn causes cartilage self–destruction. What causes this to happen, what part this plays, and when and how the system is turned on in degenerative arthritis is not yet known. Control of these mechanisms may prevent progression or halt the onset of DJD.

According to Brandt[11] a number of changes occur in DJD cartilage including:

1. Decreased proteoglycan and PG aggregation
2. A change in the GAG structure
3. Change in collagen from type II to type I

The development of osteoarthritis simulates a battle between the attempts of repair following by a failure in the system. Early on, proteoglycan and collagen synthesis is markedly increased but as the disease progresses, synthesis seems to fall off and stop. Water content also increases early on, but decreases late in the disease probably due to the hydrophylic (water binding) properties of normal proteoglycans (PGs) and collagen structure. The eventual loss of PGs causes stiffness and more susceptibility to mechanical disruption.

Primary osteoarthritis is a disease without known etiology, although there may be a genetic predisposition. Wear and tear causing subchondral microfractures may lead to DJD in this situation.

Diseases frequently associated with secondary DJD include:

Neuropathic diseases
  Diabetes

Syphilis
Aging
Obesity
Joint incongruity
   Congenital
   Traumatic
Postinflammatory DJD (after "burned out" inflammatory arthritis)
Crystal deposition diseases
   Hydroxyapetite
   Calcium pyrophosphate deposition disease (CPDD)

In summary, the biochemical, cellular, and physiologic abnormalities in DJD are just beginning to be studied. Certain underlying diseases may cause DJD and should be diagnosed and eliminated if possible. Both the inflammatory and metabolic pathways of cartilage destruction must be addressed if the disease is to be prevented and/or retarded. Pain control is helpful to the patient. Biomechanical and structural defects must be corrected once joint damage has occurred with resultant periarticular problems.

OTHER REPRESENTATIVE RHEUMATIC DISEASES

The general principles discussed with rheumatoid and osteoarthritis are helpful and may be applied in other diseases. Some of the mechanisms are operative in many diseases.

For instance, it was noted that in rheumatoid arthritis the neutrophil phagocytizes the immune complex made up of IgG, rheumatoid factor, and complement. It then regurgitates its lysosomal enzymes causing articular damage. The same mechanism occurs in other diseases. In the crystal arthropathies the sodium urate crystal (gout), the calcium pyrophosphate crystal (pseudogout), and the hydroxyapetite crystal (Milwaukee shoulder) are phagocytized by neutrophils with the same and results. These crystals are rendered appetizing to neutrophils and the neutrophils are brought into the area by various fluid phase proteins. Thus similar treatments of the anti-inflammatory reaction (pharmacologic and/or physical)—which also slow the neutrophils ability to appear at the site of the particle, prevent phagocytosis, and inhibit the egress of lysosomal enzymes—should help this acute reaction. Other measures are needed to rid the body of the offending particle that is ingested. Bacterial organisms may be ingested by the white cell also and cause destruction not only by damage from the bacteria itself but by the neutrophil releasing its enzymes in a similar fashion to that previously described.

In bacterial infections apppropriate antibiotics are needed to rid the body of the particle. In gout, the sodium urate crystal is caused either by increased production or decreased renal excretion of urate. Drugs such as allopurinal, which inhibits the production of uric acid, or probenecid, which hastens the renal excretion of the acid, are needed. The choice is determined on the basis of the individual's kidney function, measured urinary excretion of uric acid, and the extent of disease.

Patients with pseudogout often have underlying diseases which affect calcium metabolism. If one is aware of these underlying diseases, diagnoses them, and eliminates them if possible, it will help to eliminate the calcium pyrophosphate deposition. These diseases predisposing people to the problem include the following:

1. Hyperparathyroidism
2. Hemochromatosis
3. Diabetes
4. Coexistant gout
5. Acromegaly
6. Alkaptanuria
7. Neuropathic arthropathy

The cause of hydroxyapatite deposition is not yet known and remedies are not yet available.

General principles that would apply to all these diseases, however, would include rest during the acute period of inflammation maintenance of muscle strength in nearby muscles, maintenance of range of motion of the joints, and heat, cold, or other modalities.

There are a group of diseases that are inflammatory, related to rheumatoid arthritis, and yet quite different. These are often called rheumatoid variants (a misnomer), axial arthropathies (true only in some), or seronegative arthropathies (negative rheumatoid factors). Most of them have genetic predisposition as measured by the HLA locus. The HLA-B27 antigen is present in 85 to 90 percent of ankylosing spondylitis patients, the majority of whom are male. Reiter's syndrome, also a disease of males, has a 90 percent HLA-B27 positivity. In contrast, psoriatic arthritis and the arthropathies associated with inflammatory bowel disease (regional enteritis, ulcerative colitis) is seen in a normal number of HLA-B27 positive people (6 to 8 percent) unless the spine is involved. All of these diseases have a propensity in various degrees to involve the sacroiliac joints and vertebrae, thus the term axial.

Other peculiarities of these diseases include the involvement of the feet, requiring special attention to biomechanical support of them. The diseases tend to irritate the enthesis or attachment of ligaments and tendons to bones. Because of this, calcium is laid down causing spurs in the feet and elbows and fusion of the spinal column. The latter abnormalities mean that the therapist should try to maintain range of motion and posture in these patients. Other peculiarities in features and the distribution of these diseases are noted in Table 1-2.

Many diseases have systemic manifestations that require the attention of health professionals. While the physician should be aware of these problems and pass them on to the therapist, this is not always done. Some of these problems have a direct bearing on maneuvers that may be undertaken.

Table 1-2. Rheumatoid Arthritis and Its Variants

	Rheumatoid Arthritis	Ankylosing Spondylitis	Enteropathic Arthritis	Psoriatic Arthritis	Reiter's Syndrome
Male/Female	1:3	20:1	1:1	1:1	20:1
Frequency	1–6%	.05%	≤.01%	.02%	.01%
Genetic	±	90% HLA-B27	↑ HLA-B27 (only with spondylitis)		↑ HLA-B27 in all cases
Distribution	Symmetrical mostly peripheral	Axial and pauciarticular symmetrical		Asymmetrical DIP[a] and axial	
Conjunctivitis	±	0	0	0	Routine
Urethritis	0	0	0	0	Routine
Diarrhea	0	0	+	0	Sometimes
Psoriaform rash	0	0	0	Characteristic	Sometimes
Syndesmophytes		Thin, longitudinal and symmetrical		Heavy, more transverse asymmetrical	
Nodules	Characteristic	0	0	0	0
RF+	Characteristic	0	0	0	0
↓C'	Characteristic	0	0	0	0
Unique treatment	Gold, antimalarials	0	Treatment of bowel disease	? Gold	0
Synovial proliferation and joint erosions	+	+	+	+	+
Response to antiinflammatory drugs	+	+	+	+	+

[a] Characteristically distal interphalangeal (DIP), but not always.
(Courtesy of J. T. Boyer, University of Arizona, personal communication)

Table 1-3. Systemic Problems in Some Rheumatic Diseases

Disease	Representative Systemic Problems	Implications to Therapist
Rheumatoid arthritis	Nodules	Rub on clothes, splints, crutches
		Break down and get infected
	Fever, malaise, morning stiffness	Inability to comply with therapy
	Pleuritis, pericarditis	Chest pain, dyspnea
	Sjögren's syndrome	Dry eyes, mouth, vagina
		Corneal damage, dental carries
		Sexual problems
	Osteoporosis	Fractures
	Fragile skin	Easy bruising, damage
	Leg ulcers	Inability to ambulate
Osteoarthritis	Nerve compression	Parasthesia, paralysis
Gout	Tophi	Rub on shoes, clothes, can occur in internal organs
		Infection
	Renal calculi	Urinary infection, renal failure
Ankylosing spondylitis	Iritis	Blindness
	Valvular heart disease	Syncope, heart failure
	Pulmonary fibrosis	Shortness of breath
	Fractures, spine	Cord compression
Reiter's syndrome	Oral, genital ulcers	Sexual problems
	Skin rash	Problems with clothes
	Urethritis	Discomfort, social problems
	Iritis	Blindness

Table 1-3 lists a few representative problems that are of interest regarding the diseases already discussed. In addition to this, the therapist must be aware of the side effects of the drugs being used, including drug interaction, immunosuppression, allergic reaction, fluid retention, and gastrointestinal bleeding.

SUMMARY

We have reviewed in some detail the pathogenetic mechanisms of a representative inflammatory disease, rheumatoid arthritis, and a relatively noninflammatory disorder, osteoarthritis. We have focused on the complexities of the pathogenesis of these diseases but emphasized the importance of relating mechanisms to eventual treatment. Briefly, we covered some of the other mechanisms involved in other types of rheumatic diseases.

In treating patients with arthritis one must make sure of the diagnosis and focus on how the disease has affected the individual, physically and psychologically. However, without a basic understanding of the mechanisms by which the disease operates, one cannot rationally plan therapy or know what potential problems might arise. The reader is urged to keep abreast of information on the cause of the disease that he or she treats, since rapid advances are being made in rheumatology research at this time.

REFERENCES

1. Rodnan GP, Schumacher HR: Classification of rheumatic diseases. p. 36. In Primer on the Rheumatic Diseases. 8th ed. Arthritis Foundation, Atlanta, 1983
2. McCarty DJ (ed): Landmark Advances in Rheumatology. Contact Associates International Ltd, New York, 1985
3. Ropes MW, Bennett GA, Caleb S, et al: Revision of diagnostic criteria for rheumatoid arthritis. Bull Rheum Dis 9:175, 1958
4. Benedek TG, Rodnan GP: A brief history of the rheumatic diseases. Bull Rheum Dis 32:59, 1982
5. Gall EP, Gall EA, Boyer JT: Rheumatoid arthritis—Concepts in evolution. AZ Med 36:55–59, 1979
6. Cecil RL, Nicholls EE, Stansby WJ: The etiology of rheumatoid arthritis. Am J Med Sci 181:12, 1931
7. Rose HM, Ragan C, Pearce E, Lipman MD: Differential agglutination of normal and sensitized sheep erythrocytes by sera of patients with rheumatoid arthritis. Proc Soc Exp Biol Med 68:1, 1949
8. Hollander JL, McCarty DJ, Astorga G, Rawson AJ: Studies on the pathogenesis of rheumatoid joint inflammation. 1. The RA cell and a working hypothesis. Ann Int Med 62:271, 1965
9. Alspaugh MA, Tan EM: Serum antibody in rheumatoid arthritis reactive with a cell associated antigen. Arthritis Rheum 19:711, 1976
10. Stasney P: Association of B cell celloantigen DR4 with rheumatoid arthritis. N Engl J Med 298:869, 1978
11. Brandt KD: Pathogenesis of osteoarthritis. p. 1417 In Kelley WN, Harris ED, Ruddy S, Sledge CB (eds): Textbook of Rheumatology. 2nd ed. WB Saunders, Philadelphia, 1985

SUGGESTED READINGS

Hollingsworth J: Local and Systemic Complications of Rheumatoid Arthritis. WB Saunders, Philadelphia, 1968

Kelley W, Harris E, Ruddy S, Sledge C: Textbook of Rheumatology. 2nd ed. WB Saunders, Philadelphia, 1985

McCarty D: Arthritis and Allied Conditions. 10th ed. Lea & Febiger, Philadelphia, 1985

Meisel A, Bullough P: Atlas of Osteoarthritis. Gower Medical Publishing, New York, 1984

Moskowitz R, Howell D, Goldberg V, Mankin H: Osteoarthrosis: Diagnosis and Management. WB Saunders, Philadelphia, 1984

Utsinger P, Zvaifler N, Ehrlich G: Rheumatoid Arthritis. JB Lippincott Co, Philadelphia, 1985

Williams R: Rheumatoid arthritis as a systemic disease: Major problems in internal medicine. Volume IV. WB Saunders, Philadelphia, 1974

2 | Comprehensive Care

Barbara F. Banwell

In health care delivery, the concept of comprehensive care is two-fold, including both an understanding of the disease and the provision of complete care to the patient. To administer comprehensive care to the arthritis patient, the specific problems or concerns of the patient, the resources available, and the environments in which the patient exists must be addressed. The concept of comprehensive care is particularly important in treating arthritis because of the potentially wide range and chronic nature of the needs of the patient and others closely associated with the disease.

Arthritis is often portrayed as a "simple" condition, with "minor aches and pains," yet few people experiencing any type of arthritis would agree. Of the many specific diseases included within the rheumatic or arthritis category, few present single, simple, or limited problems to the patient. The effects of arthritis are almost always multiple, changing, and unpredictable, whether the condition is local or systemic, acute or chronic. Each person with arthritis has an individual constellation of physical and psychosocial needs which are both specific and interwoven. Therefore, comprehensive care of an understanding and inclusive nature is a highly appropriate and necessary style of health care management for the patient with arthritis. As a category of diseases, arthritis may well present more challenges to the health care management team than any other.

The health care system in the United States is in the process of dynamic change due to new technology, changing patterns of reimbursement, and struggles in its ethical and philosophical underpinnings. Questions such as who should receive treatment, to what degree risks should be taken, and what should be done for patients who cannot afford treatment present daily dilemmae to the health care provider. With shortened hospital stays, a fundamental change is occurring in health professional education. Since patients spend fewer days in the hospital, there is less time for staff and trainees to get to know and understand them. The accelerated pace of hospital care diminishes the time

17

available for staff to acquire knowledge of the patient's life style, support systems, needs, and resources. The physician in particular has less time to spend with the patient. On the other hand, the nurse, physical or occupational therapist, and social worker, who spend more time with the patient in the course of treatment, may gain valuable information and insight into that patient. Any person who can contribute to a matching of *needs, goals, resources*, and *action* is a participant in the comprehensive care process. The more people who understand the principles of comprehensive care, the greater the chance that such care will be provided.

The new trends in health care in America present a curious paradox. While tremendous pressure is being applied to the system to *reduce* or *maintain* health care costs, more and more *technology* is being developed for use in the health care system. The technology is not simply in the high technology equipment, such as that for magnetic resonance imaging, but in areas such as wheelchair design, positioning systems, personal products, communication systems, mobility aids, etc. Ten years ago the prescription for a wheelchair involved only the selection of size, type of footrest and armrest, and perhaps choice of upholstery. Prescriptions now must consider type of seating as to custom or standard, material of construction, type of wheel, type of upholstery, choosing from at least 10 foot and armrests, sport or utility, manual or powered. As another example, there are now at least six types of special pillows on the market for persons with arthritis, and each of the products' promotional campaigns is as believable as the next. There are several types of undersheet or mattress pads—foam, fleece, plastic, etc. No one person can be expert in all, much less a few, of these areas. *Knowing whom to call*, and then *using your network*, can enhance the information in any decision making.

Listed in Table 2-1 are a few of the organizations to be found in communities of medium to large size that might be helpful in answering questions about resources for comprehensive care. While this list is far from inclusive,

Table 2-1. Community Organizations Useful in Networking in Comprehensive Care (partial listing)

Alcoholics Anonymous	Family Service
American Heart Association	Good Will
American Lupus Society	Hotlines (various)
American Red Cross	Housing commissions
Arthritis Foundation	Kidney Foundation
Attorney General	Planned Parenthood
Better Business Bureau	Public Service Commission
Better Health Bureau	Salvation Army
Catholic Family Service	Social services departments
Co-op Extension Service	Travelers' Aid
County civil defense	United Fund
Credit counseling centers	Urban League
Easter Seals	Visiting Nurses' Association
Emergency shelters	YMCA
Family service	YWCA
Food and Drug Administration	

it can be adapted to your needs by adding those resources in your own community to it.

THE "PERSON WITH ARTHRITIS"

It is important that the "person with arthritis" not be stereotyped by health professions. We may have particular "mental pictures" of people with arthritis according to our individual practice patterns and experiences. Preconceived notions often preclude individual assessments and plans. In fact, each person with arthritis is a different individual, with special needs and resources.

Considering that "arthritis" is really a category of diseases, there are almost an unlimited number of individual situations and personalities. Each member of a group of physical therapists attending an educational meeting about arthritis was asked to briefly describe the arthritis patient who first came to mind. The following list exemplifies how different health professionals see "the person with arthritis". Among the responses were:

A 7-year-old girl with juvenile rheumatoid arthritis
An 18-year-old student with psoriatic arthritis
A 31-year-old teacher with early rheumatoid arthritis
A 36-year-old carpenter with ankylosing spondylitis
A 60-year-old store clerk with osteoarthritis of the hips and knees requiring total joint arthroplasties
A 50-year-old banker with gout
A 53-year-old social worker with osteoarthritis of the spine
A 26-year-old retired professional football player with osteoarthritis of the hands, wrists and knees
An 80-year-old woman with osteoarthritis of many years and new onset of severe rheumatoid arthritis
A 31-year-old homemaker with systemic lupus erythematosus.

The age, sex, vocation, and disease type of patients in the above list varies greatly and while each of these persons deserves comprehensive care, for some the components of care will be more numerous, specialized, and longstanding.

COMPREHENSIVE CARE VS
MULTIDISCIPLINARY CARE

While comprehensive care is often equated with multidisciplinary care, it is important to make distinctions between the two.

Multidisciplinary care or "team care" is defined by Riggs[1] as "a coordinated pattern of interaction" referring to the process as "subdividing a problem such that its parts can be treated separately by persons of different disciplines". To further define the concept of several disciplines working together, Cobble

Table 2-2. Roles and Responsibilities of the Registered Nurse in Arthritis Care

Role/Responsibility	Shared With
Needs assessment	Physician
Co-ordinate total program	Physician
Medication management	Physician
Patient education	Entire team
Direct nursing care	Others on nursing team
Casefinding	Physician
Identify financial needs	Social worker
Involve family	Social worker/physician

and Maloney[2] refine the definition further: the interdisciplinary team is a group of health professionals who meet regularly to develop therapeutic goals for their patients.[2] They stress that the *interdisciplinary* team differs from *multidisciplinary care* in that there is an effort to unify individual treatments into a comprehensive plan.

The specific roles and responsibilities of various health professionals concerned with arthritis have been described several times. At least four texts, those by Swezey,[3] Ehrlich,[4] Riggs and Gall,[5] and Kelley et al,[6] describe the activities of several health disciplines in the treatment of arthritis.[3–6] In a Delphi Survey[7] reported in 1985, the specific roles and responsibilities of six non-physician health professionals in arthritis care were detailed by three serial surveys. Included in the expert group were 10 physicians, one dietician, three occupational therapists, three physical therapists, one psychologist, two registered nurses, and two social workers. The results of this survey are presented in Tables 2-2 to 2-7. It should be emphasized that many of the activities can

Table 2-3. Roles and Responsibilities of the Occupational Therapist in Arthritis Care

Roles/Responsibilities	Shared With
Evaluation and exercise of upper extremity and hand	Physical therapist
Activities of daily living (ADL) training	Physical therapist
Recreation activities	Recreational therapist, physical therapist
Upper extremity splinting	Physical therapist, orthotist
Work/home evaluation and modification	Physical therapist, vocational counselor
Heat/cold modalities for upper extremities	Physical therapist

Table 2-4. Roles and Responsibilities of the Physical Therapist in Arthritis Care

Roles/Responsibilities	Shared With
Physical modalities	Occupational therapist
Manual therapy	Occupational therapist
Mobility, gait, posture	Occupational therapist
Therapeutic exercise	Occupational therapist
Lower extremity splinting and bracing	Physician, orthotist
ADL	Occupational therapist
Work/home evaluation and modification	Occupational therapist

Table 2-5. Roles and Responsibilities of the Registered Dietician in Arthritis Care

Roles/Responsibilities	Shared With
Assess diet/nutrition history and needs	Registered nurse, physician
Assess diet/arthritis relationship	Registered nurse, physician
Evaluate eating problems	Occupational therapist, registered nurse, physician
Define nutritional goals	Physician
Instruct patient/family in proper nutrition	Physician, registered nurse, home economist
Define and promote role to other staff	

be shared by several disciplines. The results of this survey emphasized that the person with arthritis has many potential needs which may be met by one or several health disciplines. In the term "team care" the presence of a co-ordinated group of individuals including health professionals, the patient, family, and others involved is implied. The team leader is usually the primary care physician, although the roles of leadership and coordination are certainly negotiable. Multidisciplinary care is usually perceived as being centered in the medical or health care system and as such often results in increased health care costs. Nonetheless, given the substantial loss in wages documented by Yelin et al[8] and Meenan et al[9] in persons with arthritis, if multidisciplinary care results in return to the work force or an otherwise productive life, the costs can be justified.

Comprehensive care is an extension of the concept of multidisciplinary care but includes some incisive differences. First, those who deliver or participate in comprehensive care need not be health professionals, but must simply understand the patient's needs, appreciate the contributions and relationship of arthritis to those needs and be able to supply a particular service or

Table 2-6. Roles and Responsibilities of the Social Worker in Arthritis Care

Roles/Responsibilities	Shared With
Psychosocial evaluation	Psychologist, registered nurse, physician
Assess support systems	Registered nurse, physician
Counseling: patient, family, others	All team
Teaching coping skills	All team
Educate about resources	All team
School/vocational liaison	Registered nurse, physician, vocational counselor
Discharge planning	All team
Support other members of the health care team	

Table 2-7. Roles Common to all Five Disciplines

Education of patient, family, involved others and community
Home programs
Consultation
Communication
Referral

resource. Secondly, comprehensive care may not occur in the context of complete coordination and communication, but may simply occur spontaneously in response to needs as they arise themselves. Again, the definition of *comprehensive care* is that which is given with understanding and inclusiveness.

Comprehensive care is based on, and includes, the entire community, not just the health care resources. There are endless examples of participants in comprehensive care. Among them are

Carpenters who can design and build ramps on a volunteer or paid basis

Teachers who can modify classroom work for children and adult students with arthritis

Store clerks who are willing to give extra time to the person who has special needs, including that of paying and receiving change

Commercial establishments which provide wheelchairs and motorized carts

Churches which provide transportation, comfortable seating, or bring worship to the home

Recreation facilities which are accessible and safe

Professional services other than medical which are accessible and understanding (dental, automobile, financial, legal)

Housing which is adaptable to specific problems, rather than being designed for the wheelchair user who only requires a ramp and large door openings.

Comprehensive care is based on the philosophy that the community belongs to its members and that all of its members have needs, some of which are more intricate than others. It also evolves from the philosophy that, while each person with arthritis has unique and special needs, they are very much the same as other members of the community and have much to offer that community. In summary, although an individual has primary health needs, each community has health needs, and those needs should be met by and within the context of the community, rather than by a special segment of medical services for "sick" members.

LEADERSHIP IN COMPREHENSIVE CARE

The role of leadership in comprehensive care must remain flexible according to the situation of the patient. When the patient is hospitalized, the primary physician may assume leadership or case management. On the other hand, in some hospitals a primary nurse may assume such a role. When the patient is at home and actively involved with the medical care system, it is reasonable to assume that the primary physician or other person designated would maintain leadership or act as primary coordinator. However, as the patient moves back into the community and becomes more a person with arthritis rather than a patient, any individual who understands arthritis, perhaps

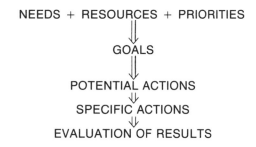

Fig. 2-1. Comprehensive care evolution pattern.

even the patient him or herself, can assume primary responsibility for case management. To reiterate, comprehensive care is based on *understanding* and has an *inclusive nature*. The case manager needs the ability to (1) assess needs, (2) assist the client in deciding priorities, (3) determine resources, and (4) develop mutual goals. At this point, potential actions can be considered and steps taken toward achieving goals.

THE BASIS AND PROCESS OF COMPREHENSIVE CARE

Comprehensive care evolves from four basic areas—*patient needs, patient priorities, available resources*, and *mutual goals*. Actions then take place (Fig. 2-1).

The determination of needs, priorities, available resources, and goals is not a static or one time assessment, but is rather one which is on-going and always dynamic. Each of these areas is subject to change at any time. For instance, the patient's abilities may decrease, needs for transportation assistance may change, a new device may suit an old need, or the goals for independence may change. Since these changes often occur when the patient is not actively involved in the medical care system, it is important that the responsibility for leadership or contribution to comprehensive care remain fluid. It may be a family member who notes changes, a close friend, a member of the clergy, or the bearer of "Meals on Wheels." A shared sense of responsibility is one factor which keeps comprehensive care alive.

ACHIEVING COMPREHENSIVE CARE

The key to organization and provision of comprehensive care after needs and priorities have been determined is the ability to *network* persons and resources. Knowledge of resources comes partially from formal training and materials, but more importantly involves human experience. In most areas, community service guides are published by organizations such as the United Way,

Social Service Departments, or private foundations. In the front of most local telephone books is a listing of community services. Pertaining to arthritis, a local or state Arthritis Foundation branch or office usually has knowledge of resources and may even have referral lists of various health professionals. Membership in the Arthritis Health Professions Association, the professional segment of the Arthritis Foundation, entitles each member to a national membership directory. Thus, if one is asked for the name of a physical therapist interested in arthritis who lives in San Francisco, one can pick up the directory and find names, addresses, and phone numbers. Members are listed by geographic area and discipline. This organization also has both regional and national meetings of professionals interested in arthritis and is an excellent mechanism for networking.

Many non-health related organizations, such as labor unions, have committees that have human assistance as their purpose. There are many civic groups who are willing to give either direct assistance or help in the process of finding resources. Although many claim that resources are scarce, in most cases they are merely unknown or unrecognized.

The primary tool of networking is the telephone, and the person trying to arrange some aspect of comprehensive care—whether it be a professional service or a ride to church—cannot be hesitant about using the phone. Some fortunate persons will have access to computer networking or bulletin board services.

In some situations a formal referral from a physician for service will be needed and in these cases the physician should be informed clearly of the service needed, the source of the service, and how the service will be evaluated. It is important that the primary physician be informed of the current components of comprehensive care in order to understand the patient's status and to be aware of the resources and service needed in the future.

CASE STUDIES

Case One—Osteoarthritis

Presentation

A 68-year-old woman with osteoarthritis, recently retired from teaching, never married, one niece living in town
Rapid onset of osteoarthritis of both knees and right hip
Lives in two-story home—had been very active with yard care, gardening, has always enjoyed travelling during summer vacations
Has Medicare with good supplemental benefits

Physical Examination

Pain on motion of both knees and right hip. Heberden's nodes bilaterally both hands, pain and hypertrophy, base of 1st metacarpal limiting pinch
Full range of motion (ROM) all joints but painful

Muscle strength good to normal except quadriceps bilaterally = Fair +,
Hip abductors, flexors right = Fair −
Ambulation painful, with severe pain on weightbearing right hip

Needs

Physical therapist
Occupational therapist
Support group
Assistance with transportation, shopping, yardwork
Environmental planning
Adaptations for recreation
Referral to surgeon
Education

Resources

Hospital
Arthritis Foundation
Handicap municipal transportation
Chore-service from home health agency or similar arrangement
Adult recreation program through adult education in public school

Priorities

Transportation
Physical therapist
Occupational therapist
Education
Chore service
Recreation

Activities

Arrange physical therapy and occupational therapy services (outpatient)
and determine time of Arthritis Foundation support and education group
Arrange regular transportation pick up
Arrange either chore service or private help
Survey available recreation services and ask them to make contact. May
also have patient contact church or alert occupational therapist of need for
adaptation

Case Two—Juvenile Arthritis

Presentation

A 14-year-old girl with rapid onset of juvenile arthritis

Last of seven children, only one in home, parents in fifties

Covered by father's health insurance, which is endangered by closing of the automobile plant in which he works

Goes to school via schoolbus—a large district geographically, bus ride is 45 minutes

Lives in rural suburbs, a few neighbors or friends nearby

Problems

Active arthritis with significant pain, fatigue

Rapidly decreased ability for independent mobility—must use toilet in school, climbing stairs onto bus difficult

Fatigue interfering with school involvement, especially long bus ride

Decreased socialization, increased isolation from friends

Fear of the future, especially with parent's increasing age

Needs

Ongoing medical management, physical therapist, occupational therapist social worker

Close interaction with school personnel, with much education about the disease and its unpredictability

Better transportation to school, adaptations to classroom

Adaptions for more independent mobility—motorized wheelchair(?)

Increased social interaction

Education of parents regarding community support systems

Resources

Physician

Home care physical therapist and occupational therapist

School services for children with disabilities

Juvenile Arthritis Association

Activities

Physician: provide adequate treatment and referrals as needed

Home care physical therapist and occupational therapist: establish home programs; use a videotape for exercise sessions; make recommendations on home adaptation; contact parent's union for construction of ramp; be available to school for recommendations regarding activity, environmental adaptations, positioning, writing equipment, etc. Also advise bus driver and others regarding transfers on and off bus

Juvenile Arthritis Association: provide support to parents and child, provide information to school via pamphlets and videotapes, advocate for family to school system

School system: adapt classroom for maximal access, enable the teaching staff and students adequate preparation for entry of child into school, provide special equipment as necessary, call in consultants as necessary

Case Three—Ankylosing Spondylitis

Presentation

A 34-year-old man
Occupation—frame carpenter
One year history of ankylosing spondylitis
Has individual health insurance policy
Divorced, three children, aged 7 to 11, pays child support and carries children on his health insurance
Former wife has custody of children, is a clerk in a convenience store

Current Complaints

Increasing back and neck pain, fatigue, loss of shoulder strength and endurance
Unable to work for more than 4 hours at a time; unable to work at all on very cold days

Problems

Pain and fatigue
Loss of work and income
Need for job retraining
Potential loss of health insurance and income; inability to pay child support
Health insurance does not cover allied health care personnel (AHP) services such as physical therapist and occupational therapist

Needs

Ongoing medical management
Work evaluation
Job retraining (or restructuring), vocational intervention, exercise instruction, consultation for a programs which can be done in a non-medical setting if possible

Review of child support—contact with court and Friend of the Court
Social support

Resources

Physician
Vocational rehabilitation
Labor union, Friend of the Court
Arthritis Foundation

Activities

Physician: give adequate treatment and make necessary referrals, discuss finances with patient.

Vocational rehabilitation: act as an advocate with employer, investigate job retraining, consider possible sources of funding for physical therapist and occupational therapist

Labor union: co-ordinate volunteer activities of union for member, offer peer support, advocate.

Friend of the Court: discuss honestly with the family the patient's physical condition, consider changes in child support or other arrangements, prevent unnecessary antagonism, mediate family concerns

REFERENCES

1. Riggs G: The interdisciplinary team approach. p. 1. In Riggs GK, Gall EP (eds): Rheumatic Diseases: Rehabilitation and Management. Butterworth, Stoneham, MA, 1984
2. Cobble M, Maloney FP: The team approach to the management of multiple sclerosis. In Maloney FP, Burks JS, Ringel SP (eds): Interdisciplinary Rehabilitation of Multiple Sclerosis and Neuromuscular Disorders. JB Lippincott, Philadelphia, 1985
3. Swezey RL: Arthritis, Rational Therapy and Rehabilitation. WB Saunders, Philadelphia, 1978
4. Ehrlich GE: Total Management of the Arthritis Patient. JB Lippincott, Philadelphia, 1973
5. Riggs GK, Gall EP (eds): Rheumatic Diseases: Rehabilitation and Management. Butterworth, Stoneham, MA, 1984
6. Kelley WN, Harris E, Ruddy S, Sledge C: Textbook of Rheumatology. (2nd ed). WB Saunders, Philadelphia, 1985
7. Banwell B: The roles of allied health professionals in the treatment of arthritis. In Gall E (ed): Clinics in Primary Care. Butterworth, Boston, 1984
8. Yelin E, Nevitt M, Epstein W: Toward an epidemiology of work disability. Milbank Memorial Fund Quart 58(3):386, 1980
9. Meenan RF, Yelin EH, Nevitt M, Epstein WV: The impact of chronic disease: A sociomedical profile of rheumatoid arthritis. Arthritis Rheum 24(3):544, 1981

3 | Physical Therapy Competencies

Carolee Moncur

Increasing pressures for accountability in health care delivery have provided an impetus for physical therapists to seriously consider their standards of practice. Society reasonably expects that health professionals be competent practitioners in their area of expertise.[1-3] The continued pursuit of a high level of competence for all individuals delivering physical therapy services has been a concern of the physical therapy profession for several years. Competence is not only the "art of being capable," but extends beyond to identify a behavior that occurs in some setting and, as the term competency reflects according to some standard.[1]

Klemp has defined competence as having a generic knowledge, skill, trait, self-schema, or motive that is causally related to effective behavior, which is referenced to external performance criteria.[4] To be more specific, knowledge can be defined as a set of applicable information organized around a specific content area (e.g., knowledge of mathematics), while skill is the ability to demonstrate a set of related behaviors or processes (e.g., logical thinking). A trait is a disposition, or characteristic way of responding to an equivalent set of stimuli (e.g., initiative), whereas, self-schema is a person's image of self and perception of the image (e.g., self-image as a professional). Motive is a recurring concern for a goal or condition which drives, selects, and directs behavior of the individual (e.g., the need for efficacy).[4]

Competence in physical therapy has been interpreted to be the individual therapist's ability to provide acceptable physical therapy services at an acceptable standard of performance. To secure this goal, in 1973 the American Physical Therapy Association (APTA) endorsed the use of competency examinations of licensure to practice.[1] As a result of a study completed by the APTA and the Department of Labor, the *Competencies in Physical Therapy:*

29

An Analysis of Practice was created, which portrayed what physical therapists do in practice.[5]

Competencies can serve to delineate between levels of practitioner expertise and specialization, and assist in achieving increased commitment to patient care.[2,6] Used as terminal behavioral objectives, competencies can define or describe what is to be learned or achieved.[7]

Competency-based education is not a new concept, having been conceived from a philosophy of education known as experimentalism.[8,9] This approach to education is based on the specification or definition of what constitutes competency in a given field. In competency-based education, time may vary, but achievement is held constant and the learner may not proceed forward in the educational process until predetermined criteria are met.[9] While conventional education is heavily teacher- or text-oriented, competency-based education requires that the learner be actively involved in the planning, goal setting, execution, and evaluation of the educational process.[10] According to May et al, competency-based curricula should be sufficiently flexible to teach both simple and complex behaviors; process-oriented—that is, directed toward what the learner will do as an outcome; and student oriented; and should integrate performance between the cognitive, affective, and psychomotor domains.[6]

ARTHRITIS: OUT OF THE MAZE

In recognition of the national problems posed by arthritis, Congress passed the Arthritis Act of 1974 (PL 94-562) and created the National Commission on Arthritis and Related Musculoskeletal Diseases (NCARMD). The NCARMD was charged to make an in-depth inquiry into the problems created by arthritis and related musculoskeletal diseases. The report of the Commission, *Arthritis: Out of the Maze*, was published in 1976 and contained more than 150 recommendations that collectively form the Arthritis Plan.[11]

In order to develop the Arthritis Plan, the NCARMD surveyed the status of arthritis activities throughout the country. The results of their inquiries indicated serious deficiencies among health professionals, not only in the knowledge of arthritis, but also in delivery of care to patients. This was attributed to several factors including the general lack of health professionals with expertise in the field of rheumatology; the need for educational programs for health professionals, patients, and the public at large; changes needed in the public policies related to chronic disease care; and the need for increased research in rheumatology. The Arthritis Plan was created to outline a national approach for the management and care of arthritis. Containing both long and short term approaches, the plan included such goals as: (1) education and training at all levels, with the initial emphasis on patients and their families, primary physicians, and those physicians and arthritis health professionals who would serve as educators; (2) the establishment of Multipurpose Arthritis Centers (MACS) and community programs; and (3) the doubling of research support for investigation of specific types of arthritis and studies in genetics, inflammation, and basic sciences.

Data collected by the NCARMD revealed a number of health service deficiencies including: (1) inadequate numbers of physical therapists specializing in arthritis patient care; (2) lack of specialized training for physical therapists and other arthritis health professionals; (3) limited treatment and rehabilitation facilities; (4) limited public health and social services; and (5) no organization that unified the resources of hospitals, clinics, extended care facilities, and practitioners to focus on arthritis problems at the community level.[11]

The Arthritis Foundation's Professional Education Committee Survey also revealed that there were inadequate numbers of specialized health professionals, due essentially to lack of adequate rheumatology programs in the educational institutions. Physical therapists were identified as one of the groups of health professionals that were inadequate in both number and rheumatology training. Questionnaires were sent to (1) the 114 medical schools listed in the *Association of American Medical Colleges Directory of 1974*; (2) all institutions listing medical residency programs in the *Directory of Approved Internships and Residencies, 1973–74*; and (3) a diverse group of institutions not listed in either of the above but known by the committee to have rheumatologists involved in patient care and/or research in arthritis. Of the 131 responses (68.2 percent) from the original 192 questionnaires sent, there were no physical therapists participating in 35 of the institutions and 81 programs, including 22 Arthritis Clinical Research Centers, and there were no internship programs for physical therapy students in rheumatology.[12-14]

COMPETENCE IN RHEUMATIC DISEASE CARE

Rheumatology Education in Physical Therapy Educational Programs

Based upon the results of findings by the Arthritis Foundation and the NCARMD, Jette and Becker selected to inquire of undergraduate physical therapy school directors to determine the level of adequacy of content about rheumatic disease care in the curricula.[15] Thirty-one percent of the responding school directors indicated that the current level of rheumatology education in their curricula was inadequate. These researchers reasoned that the remaining directors perceived their rheumatology curricula was adequate and that efforts to increase instruction time in this content area would likely fail.[15] However, according to the 1982 annual report of the National Arthritis Advisory Board (NAAB), there continued to be an adverse impact on rheumatology training of physical therapists in their process of formal education.[16]

The NAAB has generated several recommendations for curriculum content for the entry-level physical therapy program. In general, the following areas should be addressed

1. The pathophysiology and natural history of common rheumatic diseases
2. The inter-relationship of pain, drugs, environment, behavior, and activity level
3. The impact of rheumatic diseases on patients at various developmental levels
4. The methods of measurement and evaluation used in clinical settings
5. The components of comprehensive care for chronic disease, including consideration of the psychosocial aspects of the disease
6. The guidelines for referring patients and how to use community resources
7. The specific disciplinary contributions to arthritis care, with an emphasis on interdisciplinary cooperation
8. The tools for a problem-solving approach to patient care
9. Preparation for teaching (not just treating) patients with arthritis and other chronic diseases.

The NAAB further suggested that the basic entry level curriculum should be determined after a realistic analysis of the demands of clinical practice and of the health care system in which the graduates will be practicing has been completed.[17]

Development of Competencies in Rheumatic Disease

Identification of physical therapy competencies in rheumatology for entry level physical therapists, as perceived by physical therapists and rheumatologists, was completed by this author.[18] It should be understood by the reader that the 80 competencies identified by the 288 respondents to a questionnaire remain to be field tested to determine construct and criterion validity. The identified competencies are generic to physical therapy practice and are applied specifically to the patient with rheumatic disease.

The initial guidelines for creation of the competency statements were supplied by the *Competencies in Physical Therapy: An Analysis of Practice*[5] and the NAAB.[17] The survey instrument and competency questions were content validated by a panel of 10 physical therapists who were selected to review the materials because of their specific interest and clinical experience in the care of the arthritis patient. Since it was believed by the author that the primary responsibility of the entry level physical therapist is to deliver patient care, the following domains were used from which competency statements were created: (1) basic knowledge, (2) patient evaluation, (3) designing a physical therapy plan of care, (4) implementing a physical therapy plan of care, (5) patient compliance, and (6) patient, family, and community education. An additional domain called "research activities" was included on the questionnaire to ask the respondents their opinions about the entry level physical therapists' role in conducting and participating in research activities.[18]

The respondents were physical therapists (n = 208) and rheumatologists (n = 80). Prior to answering the questionnaire, the respondents were asked to consider what the entry level physical therapist should be able to do when given a patient with a diagnosis of one of the common forms of arthritis, such as rheumatoid or osteoarthritis. The complete competency statements included on the questionnaire are depicted in Table 3-1, according to the domain in which they appeared. The physical therapists and rheumatologists were to indicate whether they perceived the competency to be absolutely essential, frequently essential, useful but not essential, not useful, or not applicable for the entry level physical therapist to treat an arthritis patient.

The results of the survey for each domain are displayed in Tables 3-2 to 3-8. Those competencies indicated as absolutely essential are considered to be those an entry level physical therapist must have to treat arthritis patients. While those indicated as frequently essential or useful but not essential may not be necessary for the entry level physical therapist to treat arthritis patients, it should not be presumed that the skills are not appropriate for entry level curricula.

Some of the competencies identified by the 288 respondents have traditionally been the responsibility of an occupational therapist, social worker, recreational therapist, or rheumatologist. Unless physical therapists are employed in a large medical facility that supports a team approach to arthritis patient care, they may find themselves fulfilling the above roles. Written comments by several respondents reflected their opinions that skillful physical therapy assessment of the arthritis patient came only with experience. These respondents recommended that entry-level physical therapists should be taught evaluation techniques (Table 3-3) and encouraged to seek experienced professionals for additional consultation. Other respondents reflected that the evaluation of the patient's home conditions, recreational activities, ability to fulfill the occupational role, and work place was the responsibility of occupational therapy, recreational therapy, social work, vocational rehabilitation, and the physician working in concert with the physical therapist.

Various respondents indicated that the entry-level physical therapist should be supervised and assisted with formulation and implementation of a plan of care (Tables 3-4 and 3-5) for the patient. The new graduate should become cognizant of the team approach to arthritis care and consult with the appropriate health professional when planning. Emphasis was placed upon a well-coordinated discharge plan of care with the occupational therapist, social worker, and rheumatologist.

Enhancing patient compliance (Table 3-6) was considered to be extremely important. However, several respondents perceived that the entry-level physical therapist may have difficulty affecting this compliance. Working with a more experienced therapist may be useful in helping the new graduate gain confidence and sensitivity toward the problems related to the arthritis patient.

Patient and family education (Table 3-7) was considered to be an important skill that the entry level physical therapist should be able to accomplish. It was recommended that this activity be supervised by an experienced therapist.

Table 3-1. Competency Statements

Basic Knowledge

The entry-level physical therapist should be able to make decisions regarding screening and the need for specific evaluation techniques based on a basic knowledge of the following:
1. Pathophysiology of the common forms of rheumatic disease
2. Progression of the common forms of rheumatic disease
3. Medication regime, side effects, and speed of efficacy
4. Impact of rheumatic disease on all phases of the patient's life
5. Common types of surgery, precautions for treatment, and the process of tissue healing

Patient Evaluation

The entry-level physical therapist should be able to perform physical therapy assessment procedures on the patient with arthritis including an evaluation of the patient as follows:
1. Ambulation and transfer status
2. Skin and vascular condition
3. Neurologic signs
4. Knowledge of the disease and the treatment regimen
5. Ability to cope with the chronicity of the illness
6. Pain status
7. Swelling and/or synovitis of joints
8. Muscle strength
9. Deformity and joint stability
10. Respiratory function
11. Fatigue and endurance levels
12. Morning stiffness and joint gelling
13. Dexterity
14. Personal care
15. Home conditions
16. Ability to participate in recreational activities
17. Ability to fulfill an occupational role
18. Work place conditions

Designing a Physical Therapy Plan of Care

The entry-level physical therapist should be able to design a plan of care based upon the results of the physical therapy evaluation including the following patient information:
1. History
2. Goals, expectations and motivation
3. Pain and/or tolerance for activity
4. Deficits in muscle strength
5. Status of joint deformities (fixed versus correctable)
6. Deficits in functional activities
7. Activity of the disease (flare versus remission)
8. Potential problems which could develop due to the disease or the patient's lifestyle
9. Ambulation status
10. Ability to rest
11. Tolerance for physical therapy modalities
12. Need for adaptive and orthotic equipment

The entry level physical therapist should also be able to do the following:
1. Recognize and respond to changes in the patient's physiologic status
2. Recognize and respond to changes in the patient's ability to cope with the disease
3. Continue, modify or discontinue the physical therapy treatment and/or goals when necessary
4. Design a discharge plan of care and home program based upon the results of periodic physical therapy reassessment

Implementing a Physical Therapy Plan of Care

The entry-level physical therapist should be able to implement these programs:
1. A therapeutic exercise program for the patient with arthritis-related problems
2. An ambulation program for the patient with arthritis-related problems

(Continued)

Table 3-1. Competency Statements (*continued*)

Implementing a Physical Therapy Plan of Care (*continued*)
3. A pain management program
4. An activities for daily living program for the patient with arthritis-related problems
5. A joint protection and energy conservation training program
6. Relate the hospital and/or clinic treatment program to a home management program
7. Recommend solutions for adapting the patient's home and work environment

Patient Compliance
The entry-level physical therapist should be able to enhance the patient's compliance to the physical therapy regime as follows:
1. Determine the patient's expectations about the physical therapy treatment
2. Determine treatment goals of the patient and physical therapist
3. Design a treatment program that has simplicity in terms of numbers of exercises/tasks the patient must do and that transfers to the patient's life situation
4. Establish that the patient knows what is expected by having him or her repeat or demonstrate what has been instructed
5. Provide written instructions for home programs
6. Interpret and respond appropriately to the nonverbal message of patients

Patient, Family and Community Education
The entry-level physical therapist should be able to design and implement patient education strategies including the following:
1. Lectures
2. Leading discussions
3. Individualizing instruction
4. Programmed learning programs
5. Leading practice skills and activities
6. Role-playing techniques
7. Imitating correct behavior

The entry-level physical therapist should be able to instruct the patient and family in the proper use of the following:
1. Therapeutic exercise and activity
2. Joint protection
3. Energy conservation
4. Therapeutic electrical equipment (transcutaneous electrical nerve stimulation—TENS—biofeedback, etc.)
5. Traction
6. Therapeutic massage
7. Therapeutic heat and cold
8. Orthotic devices and supports

The therapist should be able to instruct the patient
1. And the family about the nature and progression of the type of arthritis the patient has
2. And the family about community resources available to them
3. And the family about the hazards of unproven remedies
4. Appropriately about physical/sexual problesm related to contractures, deformities, and post-operative joint replacement.

The entry-level physical therapist should be able to
1. Design and implement a community education program about physical therapy and arthritis
2. Select and refer the patient to other health professionals for treatment, education, and/or utilization of community resources

Reseach Activities
The entry-level physical therapist should be able to
1. Interpret the results of a research project
2. Apply the results of the research to patient care
3. Participate in an on-going project designed by another investigator
4. Design and carry out an independent clinical investigation to answer a frequently arising question in physical therapy treatment of rheumatic disease

Table 3-2. Domain 1. Basic Knowledge

Competency Statement	Decision
The entry-level physical therapist should be able to make decisions regarding screening and the need for specific evaluation techniques based on a *basic* knowledge of the following:	
1. The impact of rheumatic disease on all phases of the patient's life	Absolutely essential
2. The pathophysiology of the common forms of rheumatic disease	Frequently essential
3. The medication regime, side effects, and speed of efficacy	Frequently essential
4. The progression of the common forms of rheumatic disease	Frequently essential
5. The common types of surgery, precautions for treatment and the process of tissue healing.	Frequently essential

Some rheumatologists expressed the opinion that education of the patient regarding the nature and progression of one's arthritis was the physician's responsibility. The amount of education given regarding the physical sexual problems patients might have was thought by some respondents to be dependent upon the physical therapist's comfort with discussing the subject. Numerous respondents expressed doubt that an entry-level physical therapist was qualified to be responsible for community education programs in arthritis.

Numerous respondents, both physical therapists and rheumatologists, gave written responses regarding the entry level physical therapist participating in research activities (Table 3-8). These respondents indicated that research should not be a priority for the new graduate. Rather, the therapist should concentrate on gaining expertise in the other competencies, such as evaluation and treatment.

Table 3-3. Domain 2. Patient Evaluation

Competency Statement	Decision
The entry-level physical therapist should be able to perform physical therapy assessment procedures on the patient with arthritis including an evaluation of the patient's:	
1. Ambulation and/or transfer status	Absolutely essential
2. Knowledge of the disease and treatment regimen	Absolutely essential
3. Pain status	Absolutely essential
4. Swelling/synovitis	Absolutely essential
5. Muscle strength	Absolutely essential
6. Deformity/joint instability	Absolutely essential
7. Joint range of motion	Absolutely essential
8. Fatigue/endurance	Absolutely essential
9. Skin and vascular conditions	Frequently essential
10. Neurologic signs	Frequently essential
11. Ability to cope with chronic disease	Frequently essential
12. Respiratory function	Frequently essential
13. Morning stiffness/joint gelling	Frequently essential
14. Dexterity	Frequently essential
15. Personal care	Frequently essential
16. Home conditions	Frequently essential
17. Recreational activities	Frequently essential
18. Ability to fulfill occupational role	Frequently essential
19. Work place	Frequently essential

Table 3-4. Domain 3. Designing a Plan of Care

Competency Statement	Decision
The entry-level physical therapist should be able to design a plan of care based upon the results of the physical therapy evaluation. The plan should include a data base of the patient's:	
1. History	Absolutely essential
2. Goals, expectations, and motivation	Absolutely essential
3. Pain and/or tolerance level	Absolutely essential
4. Deficits in muscle strength	Absolutely essential
5. Status of joint deformities (fixed versus correctable)	Absolutely essential
6. Deficits in functional abilities	Absolutely essential
7. Activity of the disease (flare versus remission)	Absolutely essential
8. Ambulation status	Absolutely essential
9. Ability to rest	Absolutely essential
10. Tolerance for physical therapy modalities	Absolutely essential
11. Need for adaptive and orthotic equipment	Absolutely essential
The entry-level physical therapist should be able to:	
1. Recognize and respond to changes in the patient's physiologic status	Absolutely essential
2. Continue, modify, or discontinue the physical therapy goals and/or treatment when necessary	Absolutely essential
3. Design a plan of care and home program based upon the results of periodic physical therapy reassessment	Absolutely essential
4. Recognize and respond to changes in the patient's abilities to cope with the disease	Frequently essential
5. Include in the data base for the plan of care any potential problems which could develop due to the disease or the patient's lifestyle	Frequently essential

The physical therapists in this study were asked if they perceived themselves to be competent in the domains of the survey. Seventy-two percent perceived themselves to be competent, 22 percent believed they were not, and 6 percent indicated they were generally competent in these domains. The range of years of experience was from 1 to 33 years. The average number of years of experience was around 10 years. Numerous respondents expressed an in-

Table 3-5. Domain 4. Implementing a Plan of Care

Competency Statement	Decision
The entry-level physical therapist should be able to implement:	
1. A therapeutic exercise program for the patient with arthritis-related problems	Absolutely essential
2. An ambulation program for the patient with arthritis-related problems	Absolutely essential
3. A pain management program	Frequently essential
4. An activities for daily living for the patient with arthritis-related problems	Frequently essential
5. Identify and recommend solutions for adapting the patient's home and work environment	Frequently essential
6. Relate the hospital and/or clinic treatment program to a home management problem	Frequently essential
7. Select and refer the patient to other health professionals for treatment, education, and/or utilization of community resources	Frequently essential

Table 3-6. Domain 5. Patient Compliance

Competency Statement	Decision
The entry-level physical therapist should be able to enhance the patient's compliance to the physical therapy regimen by:	
1. Determining the patient's expectations about the physical therapy treatment	Absolutely essential
2. Determining a treatment program based on the mutual goals of the patient and the physical therapist	Absolutely essential
3. Designing a treatment program that has simplicity in terms of numbers of exercises/tasks the patient must do and that transfers to the patient's life situation	Absolutely essential
4. Establishing that patients know what is expected to be done by having them repeat or demonstrate what was instructed	Absolutely essential
5. Providing written instructions for home programs	Absolutely essential
6. Interpreting and responding appropriately to the nonverbal messages of the patient	Frequently essential

Table 3-7. Domain 6. Patient, Family, and Community Education

Competency Statement	Decision
The entry-level physical therapist should be able to:	
1. Design and implement patient education strategies	Absolutely essential
2. Individualize instruction	Absolutely essential
3. Instruct the patient and family in the proper use of: a. Therapeutic exercises and activity b. Joint protection c. Energy conservation d. Therapeutic heat and cold	Absolutely essential
4. Lecture	Frequently essential
5. Lead discussions	Frequently essential
6. Imitate correct behavior	Frequently essential
7. Do programmed learning	Frequently essential
8. Lead practice skills and activities	Frequently essential
9. Instruct the patient and family in the proper use of: a. Therapeutic electrical equipment (TENS, biofeedback, etc.)	Frequently essential
b. Traction	Frequently essential
c. Therapeutic massage	Frequently essential
d. Orthotic devices and supports	Frequently essential
10. Instruct the patient and the family about the nature and progression of the type of arthritis the patient has	Frequently essential
11. Instruct the patient and the family about community resources available to them	Frequently essential
12. Instruct the patient and the family about the hazards of unproven remedies	Frequently essential
13. Instruct the patient appropriately about physical sexual problems related to contractures, deformities, and postoperative joint replacements	Frequently essential
14. Lead peer-group discussions	Useful, but not essential
15. Role-play techniques	Useful, but not essential
16. Design and implement a community education program about physical therapy and arthritis	Useful, but not essential

Table 3-8. Domain 7. Research Activities

Competency Statement	Decision
Given a patient with a diagnosis of one of the common forms of arthritis, such as rheumatoid or osteoarthritis, the entry level physical therapist should be able to:	
1. Apply the results of the research to patient care	Frequently essential
2. Interpret the results of a research project	Useful, but not essential
3. Participate in an on-going project designed by another investigator	Useful, but not essential
4. Design and carry out an independent clinical investigation to answer a frequently arising question in physical therapy treatment of rheumatic disease	Useful, but not essential

terest in having continuing education, professional workshops, and seminars in rheumatology that addressed the domains of this study.

The question may be asked by the seasoned clinician regarding what constitutes an advanced-level physical therapy practitioner in rheumatology. It is an assumption by this author that those competencies identified as frequently essential and useful, but not essential can be interpreted as necessary for the advanced clinician. In a working document created by the Task Force Committee on Physical Therapy Standards, the advanced practitioner was defined as one who demonstrates unique competence and skill in a particular area of practice and continues to promote excellence in this area.[19] Since further investigation needs to be completed regarding the role of the advanced clinician in rheumatology, the Task Force sought only to offer an opinion of what this individual should be, based on their combined professional experience and Bloom's taxonomy of learning.[20,21] In general, the advanced clinician has undergone the socialization process of integrating the forces from other professional groups, the changing health care system, society, and individual concerns, as well as integrating the knowledge, skill, and attitudes related to the practice of physical therapy. This integration process has developed an individual with a higher level of professional and personal maturity, who as an advanced clinical specialist in rheumatology, can contribute significantly to patient care in rheumatic disease. In addition, this individual can serve as a role model for the entry-level physical therapist.[19]

Demand for physical therapy care of the patient with rheumatic disease is not likely to decrease as the population ages.[13,14] How services are delivered may change, and if current trends reflect future trends, the physical therapist will be required to be innovative and ingenious regarding the management of the chronic problems of arthritis. Rather than long-term "hands on" care, the therapist will find the emphasis of care to be increasingly on self-management by the patient and family. The potential importance of the physical therapist as a patient, family, and community educator cannot be overlooked. Because of the chronicity of arthritis and its effect on the patient and family, continuing management of the patient will be required. Physical therapists will need to use both their intuitive powers and training in the educational process to de termine what their patients and families need to know and do about their physical therapy plan of care.

REFERENCES

1. American Physical Therapy Association: Position paper on competency testing. Phys Ther 53:889, 1973
2. Davis C, Anderson M, Jagger D: Competency: The what, why and how of it. Phys Ther, 59:1088, 1979
3. Health Resources Administration: Competence in the medical professions: A strategy. DHEW Publication No. (HRA) 77–35. US Department of Health, Education & Welfare, Washington, DC, 1977
4. Klemp GO, Jr: Identifying, measuring, and integrating competence. p. 41. In Pottinger PS, Goldsmith J (eds): Defining and Measuring Competence. Jossey-Bass, San Francisco, 1979
5. American Physical Therapy Association: Competencies in physical therapy: An analysis of practice. Courseware Incorporated, San Diego, 1981
6. May BJ, Bemis SA, Newman J: Competency based education: Impact on practice and evaluation. Section for education: American Physical Therapy Association, Adapted from papers presented at the 1979 Annual Conference of the American Physical Therapy Association, Atlanta, 1979
7. Burns RW: Behavioral objectives for competency-based education. p. 43. In Burns RW, Klingstedt JL (eds): Competency Based Education: An Introduction. Educational Technology Publications, Englewood Cliffs, 1973
8. Dewey J: Experience and Education. Macmillan, New York, 1938
9. Klingstedt JL: Philsophical basis for competency based education. p. 7. In Burns RW, Klingstedt JL (eds): Competency Based Education: An Introduction. Educational Technology Publications, Englewood Cliffs, 1973
10. Young JI, Von Mondfrans AP: Psychological implications of competency based education. In Burns RW, Klingstedt JL (eds): Competency Based Education: An Introduction. Educational Technology Publications, Englewood Cliffs, 1973
11. National Commission on Arthritis and Related Musculoskeletal Diseases: Volume I: The arthritis plan. DHEW Publication No. (NIH) 76-1150. US Department of Health, Education & Welfare, Washington, DC 1976
12. National Arthritis Foundation: Arthritis Foundation professional education committee survey. Arthritis Foundation, Atlanta, 1975
13. National Arthritis Foundation: Arthritis: The basic facts. Arthritis Foundation, Atlanta, 1980
14. Sledge CB: Chairman's report: National arthritis advisory board. NIH Publication No. 79-1894. US Department of Health, Education & Welfare, Washington, DC, 1978
15. Jette A, Becker M: Nursing, occupational therapy and physical therapy preparation in rheumatology in the United States and Canada. J Allied Health, 9:268, 1980
16. National Arthritis Advisory Board: 1982 Annual report of the National Arthritis Advisory Board. DHHS Publication No. (NIH) 82-2481. US Department of Health & Human Services, Washington, DC, 1982
17. National Arthritis Advisory Board: Arthritis research and education in nursing and allied health. DHHS Publication No. (NIH) 80-2218. US Department of Health & Human Services, Washington DC, 1980

18. Moncur C: Physical therapy competencies in rheumatology. Phys Ther 65:1365, 1985
19. Walter J, Moncur C, Emergy M: Working document: Arthritis Health Professions Association physical therapy standards task force. Unpublished paper, Burlington, 1984
20. Bloom B: Taxonomy of Educational Objectives: The Classification of Educational Goals. Book 1: Cognitive Domain. Longman, New York, 1980
21. Krathwohl DR, Bloom R, Masia BB: Taxonomy of Educational Objectives: The Classification of Educational Goals. Handbook II: Affective Domain. David McKay, New York, 1964

4 | Patient Evaluation

Victoria Gall

Physical therapy (PT) is an essential component in the health care management of persons with arthritis.[1-3] The assessment is critical for overall understanding of the patient and for program design.

This chapter discusses the examination and evaluation of a person with rheumatoid arthritis, focusing on the musculoskeletal system and outlining other systems of involvement. Clinical features of other rheumatic conditions requiring the attention of a therapist are described in Appendix 4-2.

As is emphasized throughout this book, successful treatment requires the combined efforts of the health care team, the patient, and the family. For this reason, the evaluation and treatment sessions must be interactions, not merely encounters. The therapist must be alert, listen and respond to the questions and needs of each patient. The treatment plan must be related to the patient's goals, which will change with age, lifestyle changes, and disease process.

OBSERVATION/ASSESSMENT

Much can be learned from observing how the person enters the room and prepares for the examination. How the person shakes your hand, turns to look at you, and sits down will provide valuable information. Observing functional activities will save time, but more importantly, will allow you to personalize your later questions.

HISTORY

Although the medical history can be obtained from the patient's chart, it is not always available to the therapist, especially in an outpatient setting. Therefore, it is better to take a history directly from the patient. Essential information would be:

Age
Symptoms—onset and present
Co-morbid illnessess
Limitations in patient's terms
Treatments—previous and present
Activity level (including recreation)
Social supports
Patient goals

The time of the assessment and the patient's activity just prior to the evaluation should be noted.

MUSCULOSKELETAL EVALUATION

Baseline measurements of motion, strength, and function are necessary for designing a treatment plan, monitoring disease activity, and determining the effects of rehabilitation. Both motion and strength vary enough with age, sex, and body composition, that the therapist should avoid describing data as "normal" unless guidelines are used.[4,5] It is best to compare the patient to his or her own measurements. This can either be done by comparing the involved joint to the uninvolved joint, as in bursitis, or by comparing present to previous measurements after the second recording. This requires systematic followup, which in itself enhances compliance.[6,7]

Range of Motion

Each joint should be evaluated for:

Erythema
Warmth
Tenderness
Swelling—intraarticular effusion (bulging), synovial effusion (boggy),
        bony
Motion
Crepitis—fine or coarse
Deformities
Muscle atrophy

These findings should be measured and recorded whenever possible. The American Rheumatism Association has guidelines for recording clinical signs and symptoms, and the Academy of Orthopedic Surgeons has a guide for measuring motion.[8,9] Their values given for normal range of motion however, are average ranges and not specific to age or sex.

Active Motion

Active motion is controlled by muscle contraction. If a joint is distended or unstable, the muscles, even if strong enough, will not be able to move the joint through the complete arc of motion. The difference between active and passive motion should be documented. In addition, the therapist should comment on the suspected reason for the difference, be it pain, weakness, or muscle length.

Passive Motion

Passive motion defines the status of the joint surfaces. Besides joint incongruity, motion can be affected by the tension of the soft tissues, swelling, pain, and apprehension of the patient.

All synovial joints should be examined and joint motion recorded. Synovial tissue surrounds all peripheral joints, axial skeletal joints, and the temporomandibular joint, and around tendon sheaths in the ankle, the wrist, and the hand. Each rheumatic disease has a predilection for different joints, and the therapist can use this knowledge as an examination and treatment guide. Table 4-1 lists some of the differences.

To measure joint range passively and to test for ligament stability, the patient should be in a supported, comfortable position. Restrictive clothing

Table 4-1. Commonly Involved Joints

Joints	RA	AS	SLE	PA	SS[a]	OA	GOUT
Temporomandibular	X				X		
Spine	C[b]	CTL[b]				CL[b]	
Sacroiliac		X		X			
Shoulder	X	X	X		X		
Elbow	X		X		X		X
Wrist	X		X	X	X		X
MCP	X		X	X	X	X[c]	
PIP	X		X	X	X	X	
DIP					X	X	
Hip	X	X				X	
Knee	X		X	X		X	X
Ankle	X				X		X
Subtalar/midtarsal	X						X
MTP/IP	X			X			X

(Data from Katz W (ed): Rheumatic Diseases: Diagnosis and Management. JB Lippincott, Philadelphia, 1977.)

RA = rheumatoid arthritis, AS = ankylosing spondylitis, SLE = systemic lupus erythematosus, PA = psoriatic arthritis, SS = systemic sclerosis, OA = osteoarthritis, Gout (acute), MCP = metacarpophalangeal, PIP = proximal interphalangeal, DIP = distal interphalangeal, MTP/IP = metatarsalphalangeal/interphalangeal

[a] Symptomic joints adjacent to area of maximum skin involvement
[b] C = cervical, T = thoracic, L = lumbar
[c] First metacarpal

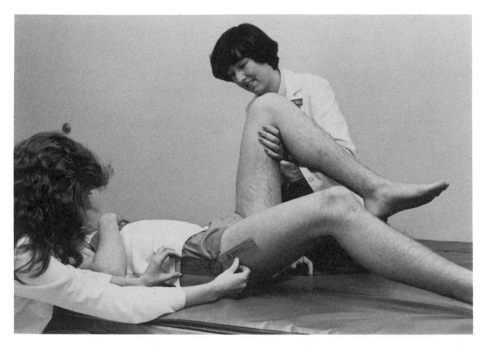

Fig. 4-1. Testing hip extension in the Thomas test position may require two therapists.

should be removed and the patient be made aware of the procedure to follow. Two persons may be needed to measure painful joints (Fig. 4-1).

All motion should be tested in a standard manner, and any exception noted on the form. Recording motion in degrees or inches is preferable to statements of "within normal limits," or "within functional limits." An example of a departmental musculoskeletal evaluation form, and an arthritis hand evaluation form are shown (Figs. 4-2 and 4-3).

The goniometer is the instrument of choice for measuring peripheral joint motion and the tape measure is the easiest tool for measuring spinal and neck motion. There are, however, many instruments available such as an inclinometer, spondylometer, and arthrodial protractor for measuring spinal movement, but they are expensive, not readily available, and not always easy to use. There are standarized techniques for measuring spinal motion and a description of these procedures and other ankylosing spondylitis tests are described in Appendix 4-1 (Figs. 4-4 to 4-6).[5] Some of the tests, however, have been modified by this author.

Cervical motion is particularly difficult to measure, so the amount of motion is frequently just estimated (ie, mild, moderate, or severe limitation). Using a goniometer or tape measure (Fig. 4-7) would be preferable with the latter technique having been tested for reliability.[10]

BRIGHAM AND WOMEN'S HOSPITAL
A Teaching Affiliate of Harvard Medical School
REHABILITATION SERVICES
MUSCULOSKELETAL EVALUATION

INITIAL ☐   INTERIM ☐   DISCHARGE ☐

Referring Service: _____ Dx: _____ Date: _____

EVALUATION KEY:

U.E. ROM Measured in: SUPINE	SITTING
(+) ROM = HYPEREXTENSION (−) = "LACKS"	(STRENGTH GRADED 0 THROUGH 5)

COMMENTS	LEFT				RANGES	DEG.[1]	RIGHT				COMMENTS
TM JOINT: (Aperture)	STR[2]	P	ROM	A			A	ROM	P	STR.	TM JOINT:
NECK:					**NECK**						NECK:
					Hyperextension	45					
					Flexion	55					
					Lat. Flexion	45					
					Rotation	80					
SHOULDER:					**SHOULDER**						SHOULDER:
					Hyperextension	45					
GH Flex:					Flexion (comb)	180					GH Flex:
GH Abd:					Abduction (comb)	180					GH Abd:
IR/ER (Add):					Ext. Rot. (Abd)	90					IR/ER (Add):
					Int. Rot. (Abd)	90					
ELBOW:					**ELBOW/FOREARM**						ELBOW:
					Extension	0					
					Flexion	145					
FOREARM:					Supination	85					FOREARM:
					Pronation	70					
WRIST:					**WRIST**						WRIST:
					Extension	70					
HAND:					Flexion	75					HAND:
					Radial Dev.	20					
					Ulnar Dev.	35					
HIP:					**HIP**						HIP:
					Extension (T.T.)	0					
					Flexion	120					
					Abduction	45					
					Adduction	10					
					Ext. Rot. (Ext.)	45					
					Int. Rot. (Ext.)	45					
SLR:					Ext. Rot. (Flex)	45					SLR:
					Int. Rot. (Flex)	45					
KNEE:					**KNEE**						KNEE:
					Extension	0					
					Flexion	135					
	Supine:		WB:		Varus/Valgus		Supine:		WB:		
					Lig. Laxity						
ANKLE/FOOT:					**ANKLE/FOOT**						ANKLE/FOOT
					Plantarflexion	50					
					Dorsiflexion	20					
TOES:					Eversion (comb)	20					TOES:
					Inversion (comb)	35					

REFERENCES:
1. Academy of Orthopedic Surgery, AOA, 1972.   THERAPIST: _____
2. Muscle Testing by Daniel & Worthingham, 1972 by W.B. Saunders Co.

Rev. 12-83

Fig. 4-2. Brigham and Women's Hospital, Rehabilitation Sevices, Musculoskeletal Evaluation form. (Courtesy of Brigham and Women's Hospital, Boston, MA.)

Brigham and Women's Hospital

OCCUPATIONAL THERAPY
ARThRITIS HAND EVALUATION

☐ INPATIENT   ☐ OUTPATIENT

Dx:_____ Onset:_____ Age:_____ _____ Date:_____ Time:_____

Referral:_____ Occupation:_____

Medications/Surgeries: _____

Prior OT/PT _____ ARA Class ___

JOINT INVOLVEMENT   Right   Left

	Right	Left
Neck		
Shoulders		
Elbows		
Forearms		
Wrists		

RIGHT HAND

		Thumb		Index	Middle	Ring	Little
	CMC		MCP				
	MCP		PIP				
	IP		DIP				

Type _____ Fingertip to Palm Crease: T_____ I_____ M_____ R_____ L_____ cm
Comments:

Circle Dominance

LEFT HAND

		Thumb		Index	Middle	Ring	Little
	CMC		MCP				
	MCP		PIP				
	IP		DIP				

Type _____ Fingertip to Palm Crease: T_____ I_____ M_____ R_____ L_____ cm
Comments:

Note the following conditions in above section.

Pain	Crepitation (Crep)	Synovial Hyper. (Syn Hyp)	Synovitis (Syn)
Swelling	Osteophytes	Dislocation (Disloc)	Ankylosis (Anky)
Nodules	Boutonniere (Bout)	Bone Resorption (Resorp)	Mallet
Lax	Subluxation (Sublux)	Ulnar Drift (Ul-Dr)	Swan Neck (S-N)

(6/80) 14-05

Fig. 4-3.   Brigham and Women's Hospital, Rehabilitation Sevices, Arthritis Hand Evaluation form. (Courtesy of Brigham and Women's Hospital, Boston, MA.) (Figure continues).

MUSCLE INVOLVEMENT	RIGHT	LEFT
Intrinsic Muscle atrophy		
Intrinsic Muscle strength		
Abd. Pollicis Brevis Strength		
Intrinsic Tightness		

TENDON INVOLVEMENT		
Flexor Tenosynovitis Wrist and Digits		
Trigger Finger		
Flexor Tendon Excursion		
Extensor Tenosynovitis		
DeQuervain's (APL, EPB) Finklestein Test		
Tendon Ruptures EDQ, EDC, EIP, EPL, FPL, FDP		

SKIN/NEUROVASCULAR INVOLVEMENT		
Skin Integrity/ulcers		
Raynaud's Phenomenon		
Sensation med./ul. nerve		

PREHENSION	RIGHT		LEFT		Comments
	able	unable	able	unable	
Full Grip					
Palmar Grip					
Lateral Pinch					
2 Pt. Pinch					

Morning Stiffness _____

ADL STATUS _____

_____

_____

MAIN FUNCTIONAL HAND LIMITIATIONS: _____

_____

TREATMENT RECOMMENDATIONS/PLAN: _____

_____

_____

Therapist: _____

Fig. 4-3. (*continued*)

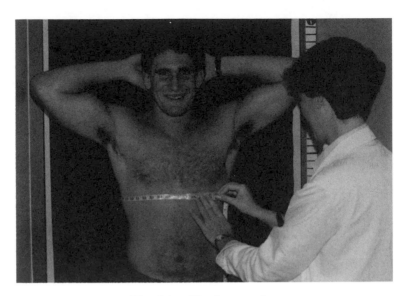

Fig. 4-4. Chest expansion.

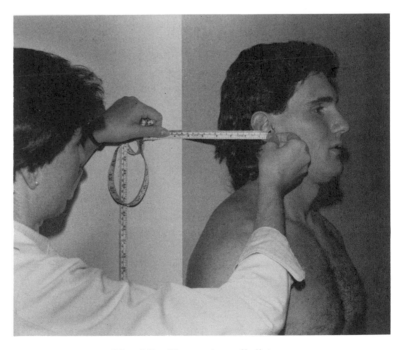

Fig. 4-5. Tragus to wall distance.

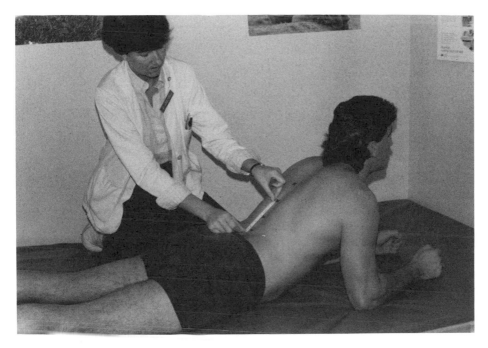

Fig. 4-6. Thoracolumbar extension (Smythe test).

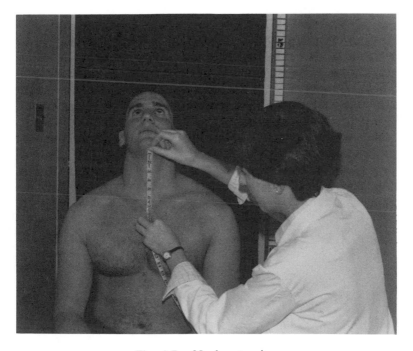

Fig. 4-7. Neck extension.

Strength

Unless testing for neurologic impairment, muscle disease, torn or injured muscle or tendon or doing a postoperative check, it is not necessary to grade individual muscle strength. Instead, it is better to test in functional groups.

Manual muscle testing is subjective and only gross changes in grade are discernable. The grading system is complicated when the patient cannot assume the testing position or has severe joint pain. Modifications to the standard protocols may be necessary. For example, the patient may need to be given resistance within the pain-free range rather than at the end of the maximally achieved active range.[11] In testing shoulder abduction for instance, a grade of 60°/4 or 60°/good, would mean that the patient could only abduct 60° against gravity before experiencing pain, but could take a moderate amount of resistance in this range. This method indicates the patient's functional strength.

Muscle strength can be measured with a dynamometer, a myometer, a torque gauge or by isokinetic testing. Isokinetic testing is not a part of the routine evaluation of a patient with a rheumatic disease but is currently being used in research settings and can be useful in following patients with polymyositis, steroid-induced myopathies, and muscular fatigue secondary to systemic illness.

Stiffness

Stiffness is described as a feeling of discomfort when trying to move a joint after a period of inactivity. Morning stiffness is a nonspecific indication of inflammation and in most patients, the length of time it persists is proportional to the disease activity.[8] Muscle stiffness can occur in diseases such as ankylosing spondylitis and polymyositis and is generally relieved with exercise, activity, or a warm bath. Muscle stiffness may also be a symptom of overuse as in repetitive athletics or heavy manual tasks.

Pain

Pain, although subjective, should be assessed for each motion and for specific activities. Pain at rest and with motion is suggestive of an inflammatory process. Pain, with motion only, is generally related to a mechanical disorder.[12]

Descriptive pain scales are often used whereby the patient describes pain as being none, mild, moderate, or severe. Visual analog scales or graphic rating scales are thought to be better methods for recording amount of pain or pain relief.[13] The patient indicates the amount of pain on a 10-cm line with boundaries. The scale may have a numerical guide (0 to 10) making it easier to respond to amount of pain. Zero indicates no pain and 10 represents severe pain. Interval use of a pain scale is a feedback mechanism for the patient.

Pain must be controlled in order to facilitate physical therapy and daily

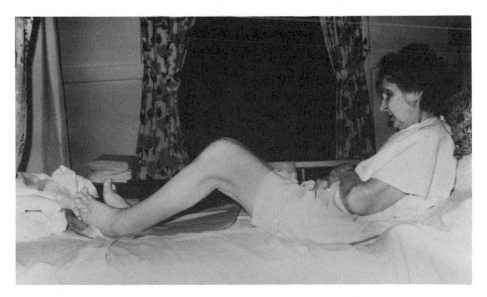

Fig. 4-8. Fixed contractures due to poor positioning.

activities. Pain coupled with capsular distension from synovitis can further inhibit muscle contraction.[14,15] Avoidance of pain is normal. For a person with arthritis, this generally implies assuming a comfortable flexed position of the painful joints and is most commonly seen in the elbows, hips, and knees. Soft tissue contractures if not treated, can become fixed contractures which are functionally disabling especially when in the hips and knees (Fig. 4-8).

Table 4-2. Common Peripheral Joint Deformities in Rheumatoid Arthritis

Joint	Position of Contracture or Deformity
Shoulder	Adduction, internal rotation contracture
Elbow	Flexion pronation contracture → deformity
Wrist/Carpal	Radial deviation, volar subluxation
MCP/PIP/DIP	MCP ulnar drift, swan neck deformity, boutonnière deformity, mallet deformity, rheumatoid thumb deformity[a]
Hip	Flexion contracture → deformity, adduction contracture, leg length discrepancy—soft tissue or bony
Knee	Flexion contracture → deformity, patella subluxation, genu varus/genu valgus
Ankle	Plantar flexion contracture
Subtalar/Midtarsal	Pronation
MTP/IP	Lateral subluxation, hallux valgus → rigidus, hammer toes/cock-up toes

[a] Nalebuff classification according to joint of initial involvement.

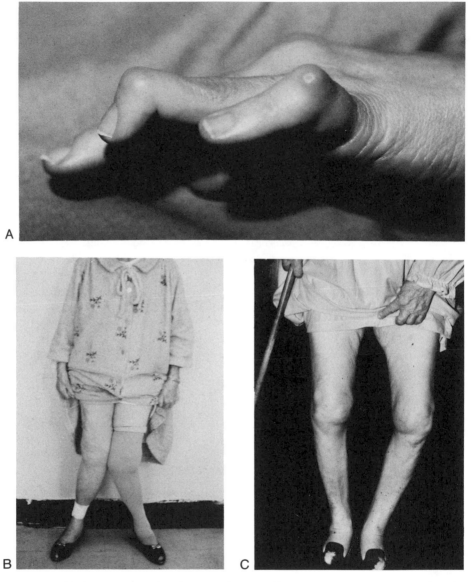

Fig. 4-9. (A) Swan neck deformity of the fourth finger and "boutonnière" deformity of the fifth finger with nodule over the interphalangeal joint. (B) Genu valgus. (C) Genu varus. (Courtesy of Barry Simmons, M.D. Dept. of Orthopedics, Brigham Women's Hospital, Boston, MA.)

Permanent joint deformities develop from long standing synovitis, inactivity, and destruction of articular cartilage. Some of the frequently seen and easily recognizable deformites are listed in Table 4-2 and illustrated in Figure 4-9. Early intervention with positioning, maintenance of motion, and strengthening of the antagonist muscles are necessary for preventing or at least minimizing deformities.

CUTANEOUS MANIFESTATIONS

Most skin lesions seen with a rheumatic disease are due to the systemic nature of the specific disease, are the results of vascular insufficiency, or are side-effects of a medication. All cutaneous changes require special attention because their presence may affect hand placement during the evaluation and positioning during treatment and may necessitate adaptions to activities of daily living (ADL) and ambulatory equipment. Cutaneous features that may be seen include:

Rashes
Decreased skin elasticity
Subcutaneous nodules
Paper-thin skin with subcutaneous hemorrhages
Psoriasis
Calluses
Ulcerations
Raynaud's phenomenon
Trophic changes

NEUROLOGIC MANIFESTATIONS

When sensory or motor impairment is noted, neurologic involvement should be suspected. The inflammatory process can affect the central nervous system as in lupus and vasculitis, as well as the peripheral nervous system.

Entrapment neuropathies are the most commonly seen problems. "Compression can occur at any point where a peripheral nerve passes through an opening in fibrous tissue or through an osseous fibrous canal."[17] Synovitis can compress the median nerve in the carpal tunnel, the ulnar nerve at the medial epicondyle, and the posterior tibial nerve in the tarsal tunnel.

Special attention must be given to the examination of the cervical spine. Prolonged synovitis at the atlantoaxial articulation can lead to instability and myelopathies. For this reason, flexion measurements are only taken actively, and flexion exercises are contraindicated for any patient with cervical spine involvement.

FUNCTIONAL ASSESSMENT

A person's functional abilities are dependent upon a number of "physiologic variables, psychosocial (e.g., coping skills, motivation, family supports, economic status) and environmental factors (e.g., transportation adaptive devices)."[18] In therapy, the physiologic needs form the basis of treatment.

Activities of Daily Living

Data from the physical examination will only indicate if the patient has the ability (motion, strength) to perform daily tasks. Instruments testing ADL must be simple to administer, meaningful, and sensitive to change. Just knowing whether a task is possible is not enough. The therapist should inquire as to the method in which the activity is done. That is, the amount of help needed from a person or a device, the amount of pain, and the amount of difficulty doing each task. There are numerous ADL scales and the Functional Status Index is an example of a self-report assessment that measures function in the dimensions of dependence, pain, and difficulty.[19] Observing an activity is preferable but even this will not show how the task is done at home or in the work environment. Being aware of this will prompt more detailed questions such as "How high is your bed?" A home visit is suggested for the patient who is experiencing extreme difficulty in the clinic setting or for the patient who appears to be rapidly losing function. Home health agencies are valuable resources both to the patient and to the therapist who does not have the opportunity to make the home visits.

It is unlikely that a standard ADL assessment or even a departmental form will include all areas or tasks that are meaningful to all patients. For instance, activities (recreational, sexual, vocational) important to a young man with ankylosing spondylitis may not be as important to the elderly homebound man with rheumatoid arthritis. It is recommended that the therapist ask patients to specify activities that are of particular importance and those with which they are having difficulty. When functional assessments are administered by the occupational therapist (OT), it is vital that the OT and physical therapist (PT) share the information and plan the treatment together.

Unfortunately time is not always available for a complete workup, but only for treating the problem for which the patient was referred. In these cases, a brief screening is recommended to elucidate other areas of potential problems. The form in Table 4-3 is a useful clinical tool, which has proved valuable in identifying functional problems in homebound elderly persons.[20]

Gait

Gait and posture analyses can be considered a part of the functional assessment. Areas needing close inspection are body alignment and joint positioning throughout all phases of gait. The patient should be observed with and

Table 4-3. Screening For Functional Disability (Rhythm, Pain, Ability)

Landmarks	Musculoskeletal Areas Tested	Self-Care Area Affected
Touch first metacarpal phalangeal joint to top of head	Shoulder abduction, flexion, external rotation, elbow flexion	Face, neck hair, oral hygiene, feeding, dressing
Touch waist in back	Shoulder internal rotation	Dressing
Place palm of hand to contralateral trochanter	Wrist flexion	Perineal care
Touch fingers to palmar crease[a]	Small joints, flexion	Grip
Touch index finger pad to thumb pad	Opposition of thumb, finger abduction	
Sitting, touch toe of shoe	Back, hip, knee flexion, elbow, extension	Lower extremity dressing
Get up from chair without using hands[b]	Hip girdle strength, quadriceps strength	Transfer ability
Stand unassisted, step over 6-in block, gait	Hip, knee, ankle, subtalar flexion and extension, small joints of feet, quadriceps strength	Walking, stairs

[a] If abnormal, test grip strength; lateral pinch strength is last to go
[b] If abnormal, test ability to get up from bed
(Liang MH, Gall VG, Partridge AJ, Eaton H: Functional disability in homebound patients. J Fam Pract 17(3): 429. © 1983. Reprinted by permission of Appleton & Lange.)

without supports and viewed from all angles. Gait analysis tapes specific to arthritis are available and Chapter 7 details the research in this area.

Endurance

The person's ability to perform physiologic work is dependent not only on the action of the muscles and joints, but on metabolism and the condition of the cardiovascular and respiratory systems. There is growing interest in aerobic conditioning for patients with rheumatic diseases. Clinicians should remain cautious about starting patients on aerobic programs unless they are familiar with the research in this area. The few studies to date in small numbers of stable patients with rheumatoid arthritis, osteoarthritis, systemic lupus erythematosus, scleroderma, and juvenile arthritis, indicate that exercise tolerance testing was well tolerated. Improvements in aerobic capacity were noted in the patients that underwent strictly monitored conditioning programs. The numbers of patient studies are too small to make any standard recommendations, but the data are encouraging.[21–23]

CONCLUSION

Patients with systemic rheumatic diseases usually account for only a small percent of the caseload of a physical therapist, unless the practice specializes in rheumatology. On the other hand, patients with soft tissue rheumatism make up a large percent. In this category are the patients with bursitis, tendonitis, fibrositis, acute and chronic cervical and lumbar strains, and other conditions with symptoms of pain and stiffness. Treatment of these conditions should always be directed at the cause and not merely the symptoms. Therefore, a complete evaluation is necessary.

The treatment of a person with a chronic disease does not end when the patient leaves the clinic or when the home exercise session is done. Management is ongoing, frequently requiring changes in regimen. In order for our rehabilitation suggestions for exercise, rest, and the use of equipment to be incorporated, they must be appropriate for the present symptoms. Therefore followup and tailoring are essential for compliance.

REFERENCES

1. Hyde S: Physiotherapy in Rheumatology. Blackwell Scientific Publications, London, 1980
2. Calin A: Ankylosing Spondylitis. p. 993. In Kelley WN, Harris ED, Ruddy S, Sledge CB, (eds): Textbook of Rheumatology. WB Saunders, Philadelphia, 1985
3. Simon L, Blotman F: Exercise therapy and hydrotherapy in the treatment of rheumatic diseases. In Woolf D (ed): Rehabilitation in Rheumatic Disease. Clin Rheum Dis 7:337, 1981
4. Clarke GR, Willis LA, Fish WW, Nichols JR: Preliminary studies in measuring range of motion in normal and painful stiff shoulders. Rheum Rehab 14:39, 1975
5. Wright V, Moll JMH: Seronegative Polyarthritis. North-Holland Publishing Company, Amsterdam, 1975
6. Parker LB, Bender LF: Problems of home treatment in arthritis. Arch Phys Med Rehabil 6:392, 1957
7. Dunbar JM, Marshall GD, Hovell MF: Behavioral strategies for improving compliance. p. 185. In Haynes RB, Taylor DW, Sackett DL (eds): Compliance in Health Care. Johns Hopkins University Press, Baltimore, 1979
8. Glossary Committee, American Rheumatism Association: Dictionary of the Rheumatic Diseases, Vol. 1: Signs and Symptoms. Contact Associates International, New York, 1982
9. American Academy of Orthopedic Surgeons: Joint Motion, Methods of Measuring and Recording. AAOS, Chicago, 1965
10. Hsieh CY, Yeung BW: Active neck motion measurements with a tape measure. J Ortho Sports Physic Ther 8:88, 1986
11. Melvin JL: Rheumatic Diseases—Occupational Therapy and Rehabilitation. 2nd ed. FA Davis, Philadelphia, 1982
12. Michet CH, Hunder GG: Examination of the Joints. p. 369. In Kelley WN, Harris ED, Ruddy S, Sledge CB (eds): Textbook of Rheumatology. WB Saunders, Philadelphia, 1985
13. Huskisson EC: Assessment for clinical trials. In Jayson MIV (ed): Diagnosis and Assessment. Clin Rheum Dis 2:37, 1976
14. Stokes M, Young A: Investigation of quadriceps inhibition: Implication for clinical practice. Physiotherapy 70:425, 1984
15. Navarro AH: Knee pain and quadriceps atrophy. p. 352. In Riggs GK, Gall EP

(eds): Rheumatic Diseases: Rehabilitation and Management. Butterworth (Publishers), Boston, 1984

16. Nalebuff EA, Philips CA: Rheumatoid thumb. p. 681. In Hunter J, Schneider L, Mackin E, Callahan A (eds): Rehabilitation of the Hand. CV Mosby, St Louis, 1984
17. Nakano KK: Entrapment neuropathies. p. 1754. In Kelley WN, Harris ED, Ruddy S, Sledge CB (eds): Textbook of Rheumatology. WB Saunders, Philadelphia, 1985
18. Liang MH, Jette AM: Measuring functional ability in chronic arthritis. Arthritis Rheum 24:80, 1980
19. Jette AM: Functional capacity evaluation: An empirical approach. Arch Phys Med Rehabil 61:85, 1980
20. Liang MH, Gall V, Partridge A, Eaton H; Management of functional disability in homebound patients. J Fam Pract 17:429, 1983
21. Harkcom TM, Lampman RM, Banwell BF, Castor CW: Therapeutic value of graded aerobic exercise training in rheumatoid arthritis. Arthritis Rheum 28:32, 1985
22. Robb-Nicholson et al: Psychophysiologic determinants of fatigue in system lupus erythematosus. Br J Rheumatology 24:110A, 1985
23. Jasso MS, Protas EJ, Giannini EH, Brewer EJ: Assessment of physical work capacity (PWC) in juvenile rheumatoid arthritis patients and healthy children. Arth Rheum (Suppl.)29 S75, 1986
24. Rodnan G, Schumacker HR (eds): Primer on the Rheumatic Diseases. 8th ed. Arthritis Foundation, American Rheumatism Association, Atlanta, 1983
25. Katz W: Ankylosing Spondylitis. p. 520. In Katz W (ed): Rheumatic Diseases: Diagnosis and Management. JB Lippincott, Philadelphia, 1977
26. Moskowitz RN: Osteoarthritis and traumatic conditions. p. 580. In Katz W (ed): Rheumatic Diseases: Diagnosis and Management. JB Lippincott, Philadelphia, 1977

APPENDIX 4-1

Ankylosing Spondylitis: Suggested Techniques for Evaluating Mobility

Modified Schober's Test[a]

Purpose: Anterior lumbar flexion

Landmarks: With the patient standing erect and feet shoulder width apart, place a mark over the lumbosacral junction; which is located between the PSISs. Place another mark 10 cm up, and 5 cm down from the original mark.

Action: Patient bends forward and reaches toward the floor. Measure the distraction distance between the upper and lower mark. Subtract 15 cm from this measurement.

NB: Thoraco-lumbar motion can also be measured by marking further 10 cm intervals.

Modified Smythe's Test (skin contraction technique)[b]

Purpose: Thoraco-lumbar extension

Landmarks: After marking the lumbosacral junction, the patient maximally bends forward and three marks are placed on the spine at 10 cm intervals.

Action: Patient attempts to fully extend spine from the prone position by pushing up on forearms. The ASISs must remain in contact with the mat. Measure the three segments and subtract the new distance from the original 10 cm.

Lateral Spinal Flexion[c]

Purpose: thoraco-lumbar lateral mobility

Landmarks: Patient undressed to the waist, standing erect with arms at sides and feet shoulder-width apart. Place marks on both sides of the lateral trunk.

The upper mark is in line with the xiphisternal junction and the other in line with the highest point of the iliac crest. Measure this distance.

Action: Patient bends sideways sliding hand down leg. Be sure the patient does not elevate the shoulder, bend forward, or flex the knees. Measure the distraction of the two points, and subtract the original number from it.

NB: Left lateral flexion is measured on the right and visa versa.

Chest Expansion[d]

Purpose: Costal-vertebral and costal-sternal mobility

Landmarks: Patient is undressed to the waist with hands on head and arms in the frontal plane. Place tape measure around the chest at the level of the 4th intercostal space of the xiphisternal junction.

Action: Patient inhales and a measurement is taken at the height of inspiration, and again at complete expiration. Subtract the expiration measurement from the inspiration.

Trunk Rotation[e]

Purpose: Objective measurement of thoraco-lumbar rotation is difficult. This test only estimates the amount of motion.

Landmarks: Patient sitting with arms folded across chest. Place marks on the posterior clavicular prominences and on the greater trochanters.

Action: Patient rotates trunk and the measurement is taken across the back. The buttocks should remain in contact with the seat.

NB: For rotation to the right the tape reaches from the left clavicle to the right greater trochanter and visa versa.

Tragus to Wall Distance

Purpose: Posture check

Landmarks: Patient standing with shoes off, heels against wall, and feet shoulder-width apart. Head should be level and hips and knees as straight as possible. Locate the tragus which is the cartilaginous posterior projection of the ear.

Action: Ask the patient to stand as tall as possible. Using a ruler or a tape, measure the distance from the tragus to the wall. If the head is rotated, measure both sides. Also record if the head touches the wall.

NB: height can also be measured in this position.

Finger to Floor

Purpose: Spine and hamstring flexibility

Landmarks: Patient with shoes off, and feet shoulder-width apart.

Action: Patient bends forward reaching to the floor keeping knees straight. Measure the distance from the middle finger to the big toe.

Thomas Test

Purpose: To measure hip flexion contractures.

Landmarks: Patient supine. Position the goniometer over the hip joint with the stationary arm parallel to the spine.

Action: Patient flexes both knees toward the chest until the pelvis begins to rock. Patient is instructed to hold one leg flexed in this position while the therapist passively extends the other hip. The measurement is recorded at the point when the ASIS begins to tilt forward, or when the flexed hip moves. Two person may be necessary for this test.
NB: Record if the test is done with the knee flexed or extended (rectus femoris or iliospoas tightness).

Intermalleolar Straddle

Purpose: This test can be done when hip abduction is too limited to be accurately measured with a goniometer.

Landmarks: Place marks on the medial malleoli or the medial femoral condyles when genu valgus/varus is severe.

Action: Patient's legs are abducted as far as possible. Measure the distance between the landmarks. Hips must remain in neutral rotation and the pelvis in a posterior tilt.

Cervical Range of Motion[f]

Landmarks: Place marks on the tip of the chin, the sternal notch, the tip of both acromia, and on both tragus

Action: The patient should actively perform the following movements and the distance between the landmarks measured

Flexion	Chin	→ Sternal notch
Extension	Chin	→ Sternal notch
Rotation	Chin	→ Acromium process
Lateral flexion	Tragus	→ Acromium process

[a] Macrae IF, Wright V: Measurement of back movement. Ann Rheum Dis 28:584, 1969.

[b] Miller BH, Smythe HA, Goldsmith CH: Measurement of spinal mobility in the sagittal plan: New skin contraction technique compared with established methods. J Rheumatol 11:507, 1984.

[c] Moll JMH, Liyange SP, Wright V: An objective clinical method to measure lateral spinal flexion. Rheum Phys Med 11:293, 1972.

[d] Moll JMH, Wright V: An objective clinical study of chest expansion. Ann Rheum Dis 31:1, 1972.

[e] Frost M, Stuckey S, Small LA, Dorman G: Reliability of measuring trunk motions in centimeters. Phys Ther 62:1431, 1982.

[f] Hsieh CY, Yeung BW: Active neck motion measurements with a tape measure. J Ortho Sports Phys Ther 8:88, 1986.

APPENDIX 4-2

Clinical Features of Various Rheumatic Conditions

The clinical features listed with the following rheumatic conditions are by no means exclusive to that disease, nor are the lists inclusive of all characteristics. The features have implications to physical therapy treatment. Please refer to rheumatology texts, and to the Arthritis Foundation's *Primer on the Rheumatic Disease* for complete information on diagnosis, pathology, and clinical manifestations.

Systemic sclerosis (scleroderma) is a generalized connective tissue disease characterized by inflammation, fibrosis, and degeneration of the skin and internal organs, especially the esophagus, kidneys, and lungs.[24]

Insidious swelling of the digits→thick, taut skin especially over the small joints of the hands, face, and neck
Raynaud's phenomenon
Nonerosive polyarthritis
Microstomia, dysphagia
Decreased secretory function
Restrictive ventilatory disease

Polymyositis is an inflammatory disease of striated muscle. When the skin is involved, it is referred to as *dermatomyositis*.[24]

Acute = swollen tender muscles
Subacute = symmetrical proximal muscle weakness
Arthralgia
Dysphagia

Malaise
Coexistant malignancy

Systemic lupus erythematosus (SLE) is a disorder in which there is inflammation of both small and medium size blood vessels in many of the organ systems.[24]

Fatigue
Photosensitivity
Myalgias, arthralgias
Steroid myopathies, avascular necrosis
Depression, neuropsychiatric disorders

Ankylosing spondylitis (AS) is an inflammatory joint disease with a predilection for the axial skeleton and proximal limb joints. It is strongly associated with the genetic marker HLA-B27 and runs a variable course that differs in severity and location in men and women.[25]

Onset between second and fourth decade
Delayed diagnosis because frequently thought to be chronic low back pain.
Stiffness relieved by exercise
Enthesopathies

Osteoarthritis, or degenerative joint disease, (OA, DJD) is a progressive biomechanical problem affecting articular cartilage. A localized soft tissue inflammation may occur around the affected joint. OA can develop at any age secondary to trauma, joint abnormality, or metabolic disease but is largely seen in the older population as a result of normal cartilage wear.[26]

Unilateral or bilateral involvement particularly in weight-bearing joint and in the spine
Pain alleviated by rest and or supportive devices
Muscle spasms, weakness and joint contractures develop from pain and inactivity

5 | Exercise for Arthritis

Barbara F. Banwell

Exercise is well recognized as an essential component of the long term management of all types of arthritis.[1–4] Therapeutic exercise may be defined as the purposeful use of the body in order to correct an impairment, improve musculoskeletal function, or maintain well-being. There is a paradox in the association of exercise with arthritis: while proper exercise is therapeutic in the management of arthritis, improper exercise may cause at least one form of arthritis—secondary osteoarthritis—and may exacerbate the symptoms and pathologic processes in any form of arthritis.

The biomechanical principles of various joint tissues such as articular cartilage, bone, ligament, and muscle are well documented. All of these tissues are affected by arthritis and influenced by exercise. Biological soft tissue remodels over time in response to increased or decreased mechanical loading, as occurs in exercise or joint immobilization. The therapeutic use of exercise in arthritis is based upon the assumption that bone, ligament, and muscle change in size and alter material properties as a function of the amount and magnitude of tissue use. The condition of the tissue is closely related to the dynamic interaction between positive tissue remodelling due to use and tissue decay due to disease or disuse. Therefore, the proper choice and appropriate utilization of exercise is essential in order to provide a therapeutic rather than harmful effect.

In this chapter we focus on the various types of exercise that are appropriate in arthritis and some criteria useful in making the choice of various exercise forms. Because no exercise program is therapeutic unless it is carried out on a regular basis, we also discuss various factors that influence the adoption of, and adherence to, an exercise program.

GENERAL GUIDELINES

It is imperative that exercise goals, activities, and precautions/contraindications be based upon identification and understanding of the underlying pathophysiologic process rather than a specific disease entity. Exercise programs designed for specific disease entities may be helpful as guidelines but should not be used as "cookbooks" to replace programs designed to meet specific goals and objectives based on comprehensive evaluation. An individual patient often has overlapping symptoms or syndromes in which the features of one disease, such as rheumatoid arthritis, seem to coexist with those of another, such as systemic lupus erythematosus. In such situation, the plan for exercise must consider features of both diseases. More common is the patient with a history of one type of rheumatic disease who later develops osteoarthritis in older years or in previously damaged joints. Another implication of the concept of "pathophysiology first" is that patients do not need a definitive "label" before an exercise program is initiated. Therapists should make use of all available sources of information to assess the pathophysiology process, including the results of radiographs, laboratory tests, physical examinations, and patient reports.

Another basic tenet of arthritis exercise is that the patient must comprehend the purpose and procedure of each exercise activity, as well as the criteria for decreasing and increasing its intensity. Patients rarely interact with a physical therapist and/or an occupational therapist over the entire course of their disease and tend to make their own changes in exercise programs. If the changes are based upon comprehensive understanding and self-assessment, these changes may be appropriate. One very important concept the patient should grasp is the inverse relationship of disease activity and exercise intensity. The more acute the disease process (local or systemic), the less intense the exercise activity should be. Thus, as joint or disease pathology enters a phase of chronicity or resolution exercise intensity can increase. Patients should understand the basic categories of exercise commonly used in arthritis (range of motion, strengthening, flexibility, and endurance) and their component motor activities. The more involvement patients have in the development of an exercise program and the more control they perceive over its implementation, the more likely they will be to adhere to that program.

EXERCISE CATEGORIES

Range-of-Motion Exercise

Range of motion is a major focus of exercise in joint disease. Because the health of many joint structures and their ability to repair themselves is highly dependent upon motion of the joint, maintenance of movement and range is essential.[5,6] Joint motion may be impaired by any or all of the following factors:

1. Weakening, stretching, or degenerative changes in the joint capsule, ligaments, or other supportive tissues
2. Cartilage erosion, loose bodies, or pannus that interfere with smooth articulation of joint surfaces
3. Shortening of muscles and tendons crossing a joint, resulting from muscle spasm, atrophy, or fibrosis
4. Edema of tissue which surrounds or overlies the joint
5. Loss of skin elasticity (as in scleroderma) of dermal scar

Range-of-motion exercises should be done as a therapeutic procedure for all joints that demonstrate evidence of arthritic involvement. For patients with systemic types of disease, it may be wise to include range of motion for all joints as a precautionary measure. The exercises should be done in as active a mode as possible with passive motion used only when absolutely necessary. Two indications for passive motion would be the acutely involved joint, which the patient is unable to move because of pain or spasm, and severe myositis in which active muscle contraction is contraindicated. Assistive or active exercise is preferred because it minimizes external stress on joint structures, uses the patient's own musculature and gives the patient control over the activity. When the patient performs all or part of the exercise, it serves as practice for the time when they must perform without a therapist present. Mechanical assists such as pulleys, are often helpful so long as the assistance is of appropriate force and not harmful to other joints. In particular, pulley exercises for the shoulder should not cause damage to the hands when used to grasp the handles. Other assistive techniques include "wall-walking," in which the fingers are "walked" up the wall to provide range of motion to the shoulders. In this case, the friction of the fingers on the wall provide assistance to achieve the range. Any pattern of single or combined motions can be employed as long as the patient is diligent in completing the entire range for involved joints.

It is usually recommended that range of motion exercises be done once or twice a day with 6 to 10 repetitions of each range, although no studies document the advantage of 10 repetitions over 5. A joint with either acute inflammation or infection should be put through its range only two to three times per session and then maintained in the anatomic position emphasizing extension. In this way the joint range will be maintained while the joint is rested. Many patients report that they prefer to perform range-of-motion exercises twice daily—once in the morning to "loosen up" and once later in the day when they feel more energetic and active.

The use of heat or cold may increase comfort and relaxation prior to exercise. Patients may use local applications such as ice packs or heating pads or may take a warm shower or bath. Exercises can also be done in the water and are often included in pool programs. The buoyancy of water is a great assistance to patients and enables them to focus on achieving full range.

If a patient is unable to complete the entire range, family members or companions can be instructed in assistance. In these cases, the assistants must understand the amount of assistance to provide, the force of assistance, and the amount of effort that can be expected from the patient. The patient must feel free to advise the assistant whether the motion "feels right" or causes pain.

Strengthening Exercise

Strength, the muscle's ability to do work, can be markedly affected in arthritis for one or several of the following reasons:

1. Disuse atrophy resulting from decreased activity
2. Reflex inhibition in muscles surrounding inflammed joints[7]
3. Primary or associative myositis[8]
4. Steroid use[9,10]

Strengthening exercises are those which provide enough resistance or "overload" that the muscle fiber responds with a physiologic change or increased recruitment. Such resistance can be provided in an isometric, isotonic, or isokinetic mode depending on the biomechanical integrity of the joints involved. It is imperative that the resistance not create stressful or deforming forces on the joint. Isometric exercises in which the muscle is contracted maximally without producing joint motion have been demonstrated to increase strength and are most appropriate for muscles surrounding involved joints.[11] Isometric exercises may be contraindicated if they cause pain due to increased intra-articular pressure or adverse rises in blood pressure.

Strengthening exercises are designed to provide a maximal stimulus for the strengthening response with minimal adverse effect on joint integrity. The stimulus in isometric exercise can be increased with the use of stationary resistance opposite the direction of the muscle pull if movement were to be achieved. For example, pushing the elbow against a wall will provide a stronger isometric contraction in the deltoid than simply trying to tighten the muscle. The resistance of one's own body—pushing one body part against another—can also be effective.

If isotonic resistance is used, such as in lifting weights, the procedure for holding on to the weights should not cause stress to the finger or wrist joints or other joints attached to the weight.

Isokinetic exercise can be appropriate in many cases of arthritis when joint damage is not severe, since the resistance will be varied and conform to the pattern of force production without overloading weaker portions of the range.

Strengthening exercise should be introduced as early as possible to the patient with arthritis, even before loss of strength has taken place. Muscle contraction functions to absorb impact and shock in weight bearing and optimal strength will serve to protect and preserve the joint.

Table 5-1. Physiologic Limitations on Endurance Exercise

Respiratory
    Abnormal pulmonary mechanics
    Ventilatory muscle weakness or fatigue
    Impaired gas exchange
    Decreased tissue elasticity
Cardiovascular
    Impaired cardiac function
    Decreased coronary blood flow
    Impaired oxygen delivery
Energy Metabolism
    Impaired absorption or utilization of energy sources
    Disorders of muscle energy metabolism
Hormonal
    Impaired hormonal response

Cardiovascular Conditioning—Endurance

Until the past few years, most physicians and therapists recommended that the arthritis patient use great caution in exercise programs and not participate in vigorous activity which might result in increase in pulse or respiration rate. Vigorous exercise was seldom recommended and little attention was given to cardiovascular conditioning. With the popular interest in "aerobic" exercise in the 1970s and 1980s, patients with arthritis began asking if they could participate in these activities. A 7-year study of patients in Sweden demonstrated that those patients who participated in conditioning exercises as well as the usual range-of-motion and strengthening activities had better outcomes in function, occupational status, and physical parameters.[12–15]

Another series of studies demonstrated that patients with osteoarthritis and rheumatoid arthritis could participate in a symptom-limited graded exercise test on a bicycle ergonometer without negative consequences.[16] These patients were also able to improve cardiovascular function with a 12-week bicycle ergometer aerobic conditioning program.[17] Properly designed conditioning activities that take into account the level of joint stability, pain, and other limiting factors can be very helpful to arthritis patients who are not in acute phases of their disease. Brisk walking, dancing, swimming, and bicycling (stationary or mobile) are examples of such activities.[18] These activities must be pursued with some caution because of the various pathologic processes that may impose limitations upon endurance. Table 5-1 denotes some of these processes.

Flexibility

Flexibility exercises are defined in this chapter as those that involve the neck, trunk, and hips in motions of flexion, extension, lateral flexion, and rotation. They may sometimes be combined with motions of the extremities, such as reaching with the arms or extending the legs. Flexibility is a more encompassing concept than range of motion because it includes ease and grace of movement, factors that are somewhat subjective and not easily measured. Trunk flexibility can be measured with tests such as the "sit and reach" test.

People with arthritis may lose trunk flexibility and ease of motion as a result of arthritic involvement of the spine or habitual muscle tension and splinting in the shoulder and hip areas. Pain and stiffness cause guarding and interfere with fluid, graceful movement. People with arthritis are less likely to engage in reaching and twisting activities, motions important to flexibility.

Flexibility exercises can be done in a standing or sitting position. In the early stages of exercise the sitting position is preferred because the hips are stabilized and the patient feels more secure. The exercise activities should include slow, active movements that begin in small arcs of motion and increase in amplitude as the patient feels comfortable. The patient can engage in slow stretching as desired, but ease of movement should be stressed throughout. Music can be used to help pace the exercises and maintain patient involvement.

Improvement in trunk flexibility often has direct association with improved functions such as pulling on shoes, socks, and slacks and securing buttons or zippers in the backs of clothes. Patients report a feeling of relaxation and calm after flexibility workouts and are very positive in their response. Flexibility exercises, which may be done as a part of water exercise programs, are also well received.

EXERCISE FOR ITS OWN SAKE

The most attractive exercise for people with arthritis is exercise that is done "for its own sake," bringing a variety of rewards and pleasures which may be quite personal. Physical therapists tend to be very serious about exercise, focusing on goals, objectives, precautions, and contraindications. However, this professional attitude may actually inhibit people from participating in exercise activities. Many people enjoy physical activities such as leisure walking, dancing, swimming, or golfing for the intrinsic values of expression, elevation of mood, or the social interaction that occurs simultaneously. Just as Americans tend to organize everything including exercise, health professionals tend to view exercise as a treatment. Most people will engage in any activity if the resulting rewards are felt to be worth the effort. The physical therapist should value exercise which is done "for its own sake" and not negate its outcomes because these may be difficult to measure. Therapists can act as advisors in the adaptation of activities to meet limitation imposed by arthritis, but should guard against being prohibitive or overly cautious. The ultimate of goal of exercise is to help people enjoy physical expression and feel good about themselves.

WATER EXERCISE PROGRAMS

The old adage "swimming is the best exercise for arthritis" is strongly supported by popular acclaim, if not by scientific evidence. But swimming per se, with the utilization of specific strokes and kick patterns, is not the only physical activity which can be done in the water. Almost any physical motion can occur in the water, provided there is enough room for the motion to be completed. The buoyancy of water supports weakened and painful limbs, eases motion, and provides a freedom of motion not possible on land. Water can also provide resistance which is isokinetic in nature, accommodating to the force expended. For the patient who wishes cardiovascular conditioning the jogging or other aerobic activity can be done in a pool. Thus water is an excellent environment for all types of arthritis.

Many community swimming pools have programs especially designed for people with arthritis. The Arthritis Foundation also has developed an approved and carefully supervised program led by trained instructors who meet rigid selection criteria. Leadership training for this program is available through local or state Arthritis Foundation offices.

ADHERENCE TO EXERCISE PROGRAMS

Although a considerable body of knowledge exists about adherence to fitness and cardiac rehabilitation exercise programs, very little research has been done on patterns and mediators of adherence in arthritis exercise. This is unfortunate because even the best exercise program is useless if there are no participants.

Several authors have discused the factors which characterize the noncomplier in cardiorespiratory exercise programs.[19,20] Some of these factors include cigarette smoking, being overweight, lack of support from a spouse or employer, inconvenient exercise facilities, pain or excessive fatigue resulting from exercise, lack of positive results, and boring regimens. These characteristics apply to individuals involved in a group exercise program and may not be valid for those in individual exercise programs.

Several investigators have examined personal factors that might mediate exercise adherence such as locus of control, self-efficacy, and self-motivation.[21,22] Again, few studies have addressed people with arthritis, but it is reasonable to assume that the findings might have some general implications.

Stoedefalke suggests a variety of strategies for motivating the older adult to initiate and adhere to an exercise program.[23] He suggests behavioral contracting, self-control techniques, enhancement of identity, stimulation, and attention to safety and security. A detailed program using behavioral management strategies has been developed for use in all areas of health and fitness.[24] This program includes shaping, reinforcement, control, reinforcement fading, stimulus control, contracting, cognitive control, self-monitoring, and generalization training. This type of program would be appropriate to either the group or individual setting and could be easily applied to the participant in an exercise program for people with arthritis. Many other strategies for improving adherance have been proposed.[25] Exercise programs for people with arthritis should be designed with these strategies in mind.

REFERENCES

1. Fred DM: Rest versus activity in arthritis and physical medicine. In Licht S. (ed): Arthritis and Physical Medicine. Waverly Press, Baltimore, 1969
2. Swezey R: Essentials of physical management and rehabilitation in arthritis. Arthritis Rheum 3:349, 1974
3. Calabro JJ, Wykert J: The Truth About Arthritis Care. David McKay, New York, 1977
4. Freyberg RH: Recent trends in the treatment of rheumatoid arthritis. Ohio State Med J 38:813, 1942
5. Pamoski MJ, Colyer RA, Brandt KD: Joint motion in the absence of normal loading does not maintain normal articular cartilage. Arthritis Rheum 23:325, 1980
6. Radin EL: The physiology and degeneration of joints. Sem in Arth Rheum 2:245, 1972–3
7. deAndrade J, et al: Joint distension and reflex muscle inhibition in the knee. J Bone Joint Surg 47:313, 1965
8. Haslock DI, Wright V, Harriman DGF: Neuromuscular disorders in rheumatoid arthritis: A motor-point muscle biopsy study. Quart J Med 39:335, 1970
9. Danneskiold-Samson B, Grimsby G: The influence of prednisone on the muscle morphology and muscle enzymes in patients with rheumatoid arthritis. Clin Sci 71:693, 1986
10. Danneskiold-Samson B, Grimsby G: Muscle morphology and enzymes in proximal and distal muscle groups of lower limbs from patients with corticosteroid treated rheumatoid arthritis. Clin Sci 71:685, 1986
11. Nordesjo LO, Nordgren B, Wigren A, Kolstad K: Isometric strength and endurance in patients with severe rheumatoid arthritis or osteoarthritis in the knee joints: A comparative study in healthy men and women. Scand J Rheum 12:157, 1983
12. Ekblom B, et al: Physical performance in patients with rheumatoid arthritis. Scand J Rheum 3:121, 1974
13. Ekblom B, et al: Effect of short-term physical training on patients with rheumatoid arthritis. Scand J Rheum 4:80, 1985
14. Ekblom B, et al: Effect of short–term physical training on patients with rheumatoid arthritis-A 6–month follow-up study. Scand J Rheum 4:87, 1975
15. Nordemar R: Physical training in rheumatoid arthritis: A controlled long-term study. II. Functional capacity and general attitudes. Scand J Rheum 10:25, 1981
16. Beals C, et al: Oxygen cost of work in rheumatoid arthritis patients. Clin Res 28:752A, 1980
17. Harkcom TM: Therapeutic value of graded aerobic exercise training in rheumatoid arthritis. Arth Rheum 28:32, 1985
18. Porcari J, Maccarron R, Kline G, et al: Is fast walking an adequate aerobic training stimulus for 30–69 year-old men and women? Phys Sports Med 15:119, 1987
19. Dishman RK, Sallis JF, Orenstein DR: The determinants of physical activity and exercise. J US Public Health Service 2:245, 1973
20. Oldridge NB: Compliance with intervention and rehabilitation exercise programs-A review. Pre Med 11:56, 1984
21. Dishman R, Ickes W, Morgan WP: Self-motivation and adherence to habitual physical activity. J App Soc Psych 10:115, 1980
22. Beck KH, Lund AK: The effects of health threat seriousness and personal efficacy upon intentions and behavior. J App Soc Psych 11:401, 1981

23. Stoedefalke KG: Motivating and sustaining the older adult in an exercise program. Top Ger Rehab 1:78, 1985
24. Martin JE, Dubbert PM: Behavioral management strategies for improving health and fitness. J Card Rehab 4:200, 1984
25. Martin JE, Dubbert PM: Exercise applications and promotion in behavioral medicine: Current status and future directions. J Consult Clin Psych 50:1004, 1982

6 | Physical Modalities

Kathleen Haralson

The use of physical modalities to alleviate musculoskeletal pain and stiffness probably precedes recorded history. Primitive man must have warmed his aching muscles by a fire, enjoyed the soothing warm water of natural hot springs, and rubbed snow and ice over a swollen joint. Thousands of years later Hippocrates documented the virtues of many modalities and through succeeding centuries the indications for their use have remained virtually unchanged. From time immemorial modalities have been an accepted component of the total treatment program for individuals with arthritis.

Curiously, in spite of thousands of years of accepted use there are remarkably few studies on the efficacy of modalities. The empirical evidence on their behalf is certainly very strong. Nevertheless, physical therapists must be cognizant of the general lack of proven efficacy and document modality use through well-planned and carefully conducted studies.

The modalities discussed in this chapter include those most commonly employed in the treatment of arthritis: heat, cold, hydrotherapy, traction and electricity, specifically transcutaneous electrical nerve stimulation (TENS), and biofeedback. All can be reproduced in the home setting, usually relatively conveniently and inexpensively. To date, no single modality has been proven more effective than any other and they are frequently given in combinations (e.g., hot packs and traction).

The variable nature of rheumatic diseases and pain perception and relief requires an open, flexible attitude on the part of the physical therapist toward the choice of modalities. Furthermore the ease of application in the home may lead to abuse or misuse on the part of the patient. Comprehensive treatment should always include instruction on the safe and appropriate use of modalities.

HEAT

Heat has served as a panacea for all varieties of aches and pains since earliest man first experienced the sun's warmth. Once he learned to harness heat by building fires and utilizing the heat-retaining properties of rocks and sand he had a readily available, and more controllable, source of warmth. In the late seventeenth century Robert Boyle's observations on the constancy of human body temperature and Newton's law of the conservation of mechanical energy laid the foundation for modern theories of heat.[1] The discovery of electricity in the mid-nineteenth century introduced new artificial methods of heat application that overcame many of the previous limitations of fuel and apparatus. Historically, the use of heat to alleviate the pain accompanying arthritis is well-documented, and heat continues to be part of the total treatment program.[2-4]

Neurophysiologic Mode of Action

Although centuries of tradition and favorable clinical experience sanction the use of heat to alleviate pain, it is unclear precisely how it does so. Numerous studies have investigated the effect of heat in its many forms on skin and tissue temperature, blood flow, muscle spasm, muscle and tendon extensibility, free nerve endings, and peripheral nerves, but the correlation between degree of pain relief and tissue temperature change has yet to be determined.[5-8]

Nevertheless, heat applications produce several therapeutically desirable physiologic effects. Heat increases local blood flow due to arteriolar and capillary dilatation. Localized edema accompanies increased blood flow and internal muscle temperatures may be elevated as well.[1] Although muscle spasm may be decreased by increasing muscle blood flow, thus decreasing the accumulation of muscle metabolites,[5] some investigators question whether muscle blood flow is significantly altered.[9] Muscle spasm is more probably relieved by its relaxing affects on striated skeletal musculature, and by the direct effect of heat on the gamma fibers of the muscle spindles, which decrease spindle activity and sensitivity to stretch.[5,9-11] Heat applications have demonstrated the capacity to increase the extensibility of collagen tissue. However, to achieve sufficient residual elongation for therapeutic benefit a mechanical stretch must accompany the heat.[7] Heat may also act selectively on free nerve endings and peripheral nerve fibers to increase the pain threshold.[8-10]

The causes of pain accompanying arthritis are poorly understood and probably stem from many sources, depending on the specific pathology involved. Heat may have a sedative effect on the free nerve endings and pain receptors present in the synovium and joint capsule as well as produce relaxation of surrounding musculature. Most individuals are conditioned to expect beneficial effects from heat applications and this could secondarily relieve muscle guarding. Certainly the application of heat produces a positive psychological effect which should not be overlooked.[12]

The depth of heat penetration depends on whether the type of heat applied is "superficial" or "deep". Superficial heat penetrates only a few millimeters so that while it may effectively increase skin temperature from 40° to 45° C, it will not significantly elevate intra-articular temperature.[9] In contrast, deep heat, or diathermy, has been shown to elevate intra-articular temperatures.[13] Horvath and Hollander[14] demonstrated a positive correlation between increased intra-articular temperature and clinical activity in rheumatoid arthritis, while Harris and McCroskery[15] noted that an increase of 5° C produced a fourfold increase in enzymatic lysis of human cartilage collagen by rheumatoid synovial collagenase.[14,15] Accumulating data suggest that deep heating of inflammed joints may hasten joint destruction in rheumatoid arthritis.[16]

Ultrasound penetrates more deeply than either shortwave or microwave diathermy and the majority of the physiologic responses are due to its thermal, rather than mechanical, effects on tissues.[17] The localized thermal action increases intracellular metabolism, exudates and precipitates are absorbed, tissue deposits broken up, and edema and muscle hypertonicity decreased.[5,18] Experimentally, ultrasound has demonstrated the capacity to produce greater tendon extensibility.[19]

The primary therapeutic value of ultrasound is related to its selectivity of absorption. Heating is most marked in superficial bone, synovium and capsular tissues, ligaments, myofascial interfaces, nerve trunks, tendons, and tendon sheaths.[10,17]

Indications

The indications for heat therapy are numerous and wide-ranging. Heat is frequently applied to decrease joint stiffness and muscle spasm and to relieve the pain accompanying many musculoskclctal disorders. On an anecdotal basis heat is most often recommended for subacute and chronic conditions; if tolerated, cold is usually advised for acute inflammatory conditions and connective tissue injuries.[20,21] Heat is used for rheumatoid arthritis, degenerative joint disease, progressive systemic sclerosis, and other rheumatic conditions to alleviate secondary muscle spasm and stiffness and to increase the extensibility of contracted soft tissues.

Shortwave diathermy is indicated when deep heat for the superficial musculature is desired, and microwave diathermy for heating both superficial and deep musculature.[20] However, diathermy does not appear to offer any advantages over superficial heat for the pain and stiffness accompanying arthritis[21] and may be contraindicated[16] in the presence of joint inflammation.

The selective heating capacities of ultrasound make it particularly valuable for the treatment of joint contractures, periarthritis, bursitis, epicondylitis, and similar conditions.[10,18] Although the ability to break up calcareous deposits has been attributed to ultrasound, controlled studies have not sustained this premise.[22]

Favorable clinical experience and anecdotal evidence strongly endorse the use of heat but few controlled studies have been conducted. The vast majority of studies either examined the physiologic effects of heat or compared one method of heat application to another. Two controlled studies examined the effect of paraffin on the rheumatoid hand with inconclusive results.[23,24] In several uncontrolled studies investigators assessed the effects of heat, usually in combination with other treatment modalities (range-of-motion exercise, massage), and although they demonstrated positive results it is impossible to ascertain which modality effected improvement.[6,25-27] Thus, while heat applications do appear to offer relief to the individual with arthritis, their chief benefits lie in their use as an adjunct to exercise.

Application

Superficial heat is transmitted by conduction, convection, and radiation. Deep heat is transmitted by conversion. Conductive heating devices include the heating pad, hydrocollator pack, paraffin wax bath, and hot water bottle. Radiant heat is supplied by infrared lamps and convective heat by moist air baths or a sauna. Although investigators have attempted to assess the value of one form of superficial heat over another, the general consensus is that they achieve similar local heating and peripheral reflex effects.[28-30] The choice should depend on the specific area treated and individual patient preference.

With the exception of ultrasound, all heat modalities should be applied for approximtely 20 to 30 minutes to achieve and sustain sufficient local heating effects. Ultrasound is usually applied for 5 to 10 minutes at 0.5 to 1.0 watts/cm.[2] See the modalities chart (Table 6-1) for information on the application of individual modalities.

An additional method of heat application is through the utilization and retention of body heat. Joint warmers and elastic supports aid the body to retain warmth in addition to providing increased joint stability. Sleeping bags have been suggested to decrease the morning stiffness accompanying rheumatoid arthritis,[31] and empirical experience suggests that closely wrapping patients in layers of blankets for 30 minutes prior to exercise helps conserve body warmth, reduce joint stiffness, and promote general relaxation.

Precautions

Heat applications are contraindicated or should be used with caution in the presence of decreased sensation, peripheral vascular disease, skin ulcerations, and atrophic changes.[5,12,17,21] Diathermy should not be used over inflammed joints.[16]

However, the greatest danger from heat therapy may lie not in its application in the clinical setting, but rather from indiscriminant home use. Therapists should provide patients with accurate, careful instruction regarding home heat applications. A thorough review of the potential hazards of heat treatment

Table 6-1. Modalities

Modality	Temperature	Application	Time (minutes)	Considerations
Heat				
Hydrocollator pack/hot packs	140°	Localized Insulation necessary	20–30	Commercially available for home use May require assistance to apply Low-moderate cost
Paraffin wax	120°	Localized Dip and wrap in paper and toweling or dip and hold in wax	20–30	May require assistance for effective home use Low cost
Infrared lamp	500 + watt bulb	Localized Place several inches from exposed area	20–30	Convenient for home use Low cost
Electric heating pad/glove	100°–105°	Localized	20–30	Convenient for home use Low cost
Electric blanket	70°–80°	Generalized	20 min–several hours	Convenient for home use Moderate cost
Elastic joint supports/warmers, blankets, sleeping bags	Retain body heat	Localized or generalized	30 min–several hours	Convenient for home use Low cost
Ultrasound	.5 → 1.5 W/CM°	Localized Use coupling medium	5–15	PT-administered

(Continued)

Table 6-1. Modalities (*continued*)

Modality	Temperature	Application	Time (minutes)	Considerations
Cold				
Cold hydrocollator packs	50°	Localized Insulation necessary	20–30	Commercially available May require assistance to apply Low moderate cost
Slush pack	35°–45°	Localized Fill doubled plastic Zip-Loc bags with 1 cup denatured alcohol and 2 cups water-freeze Insulation necessary	10–20	Convenient home use Low cost
Home cold packs	35°–45°	Localized Apply slightly thawed bag of frozen vegetables or crushed ice Insulation may be necessary	10–20	Convenient home use Low cost
Ice massage	35°–45°	Localized Rub large ice cube or frozen cup of water over area	5–10	Convenient home use

Hydrotherapy

	Temperature	Location	Time (min)	Comments
Whirlpool/Spas	110°	Localized	20–30	Commercially available for home use Limited scope for exercise—distal extremities only Moderate → high cost
Hubbard tank/lowboy	100°–102°	Generalized	20–30	Broad scope for exercise Moderate → high cost
Therapeutic pool; home/community pool	82°–95°	Generalized	15–60	Broad scope for exercise Cost variable
Baths/showers	100°–105°	Generalized and low extremity/trunk	15–30	Variable scope for exercise Low cost
Contrast baths	cold = 65°–70° hot = 100°–105°	Localized feet/hands	Up to 30 Recommended times for alternative heat and cold vary (i.e., 6 hot, 4 cold; 4 hot, 1 cold; 8 hot, 1 cold; 10 hot, 1 cold)	Limited scope for exercise—hands and feet only May require assistance for home use Low costs

should be part of all home program instruction, as patients may apply heat whether or not therapists have recommended it.

Although heat is a universally accepted treatment for arthritis, it has not been shown to affect the course of disease or patient outcome. For the therapist, its clinical utility lies in its ability to temporarily decrease pain and facilitate relaxation. As such it is a valuable adjunct to exercise.

CRYOTHERAPY

Hippocrates is said to have applied ice and snow to the body before beginning an operation.[32] Cold agents were originally applied to reduce pain, fever, and bleeding but in recent decades have also been used to reduce inflammation, spasticity, and muscle spasms. Although cryotherapy is most commonly used in the treatment of athletic injuries and other trauma, it is a valuable adjunct in the treatment of arthritis.

Neurophysiologic Mode of Action

Cold applications lower the temperature of the underlying skin and tissues. The depth of penetration, physiologic changes, and speed with which cooling is achieved are directly influenced by the length of application, type of agent, and temperature and conductivity of the treated tissue. Reports in the literature concerning the amount of temperature reduction vary considerably due to the wide range of variables involved in cryotherapy.

Superficial vasoconstriction of cutaneous blood vessels is the most immediate physiologic change to occur following a cold application. Cold also acts directly on smooth muscle and increases blood viscosity, and these reactions, in conjunction with reflex vasoconstriction and decreased vasodilator metabolites, combine to reduce local blood flow.[33,34] When the tissue temperature drops below 10° C a phenomenon known as the "hunting response" occurs.[35] Vasodilation and vasoconstriction alternate to produce periodic temperature changes.

Physiologic responses to local cooling also include metabolic, neural, and neuromuscular effects. Cooling produces a metabolic effect opposite to that of heat.[36] Cell metabolism is reduced and the need for oxygen decreases. The neural effects include altered nerve conduction velocity, nerve receptor firing, and synaptic transmissions.[34] Cold has been demonstrated to alter muscle electrical activity and temporarily diminish spasticity and muscle spasms.[37–39] Some investigators[40,41] have postulated that lowered temperature might inhibit the activity of enzymes that damage cartilage and that cryotherapy might stimulate the production of endorphins,[41] but definitive evidence has not been produced to support these speculations. Although cold applications may produce desirable effects such as reduced pain, swelling, inflammation, and muscle spasms, long term applications may also induce temporary muscle stiffness and lowered muscle efficiency.[36,42]

Indications

Cold applications are commonly used to reduce the edema and pain that follows acute trauma and musculoskeletal injury.[32,43] For the same reasons they are frequently used postoperatively.[44] Other indications include the reduction of spasticity that may accompany upper motor neuron lesions and the treatment of individual trigger points associated with myofascial pain syndromes.[45] Ice massage has been demonstrated to alleviate pain effectively and increase motion for acute bicipital tendinitis.[46] Cold decreases connective tissue distensibility and therefore is not recommended for the treatment of contractures. However, if the loss of motion is due to pain and muscle guarding, cold applications may alleviate these symptoms and permit greater stretching.[36]

Although both heat and cold have been shown to reduce arthritis pain, empirical evidence suggests that cold is most effective for acute inflammatory pain and heat for subacute and chronic pain.[47,48] Several investigators have compared the two. In a study comparing heat to cold applications Utsinger and associates noted that 50 percent of the patients preferred heat, 32 percent preferred cold, and 18 percent had no preference.[41] All patients demonstrated decreased pain and improvement in sleep duration and timed functional tests. In a study evaluating cryotherapy alone for intractable knee pain in patients with rheumatoid arthritis investigators applied ice packs to one knee three times a day for 4 weeks.[49] Range of motion and function increased and pain decreased for the treated knee, with no change noted for the untreated knee. Kirk and Kelsey evaluated patient preference of heat and cold and reported that 60 percent of their patients preferred cold, while both groups noted an increase in range of motion.[50]

Clarke et al conducted a study to compare the effects of ice, short-wave diathermy, and untuned short wave diathermy on the knees of patients with osteoarthritis.[51] Subjects were assessed for pain, stiffness, swelling, and range of motion. At 3 weeks the group treated with ice demonstrated the most significant reduction in pain with all three groups showing similar improvements at 3 months. Hecht and associates compared heat and cold after total knee arthroplasty.[52] Patients were randomized into three groups to compare the results of ten treatments of heat and exercise, cold and exercise, and exercise alone. No group differed significantly from the other in range of motion but the group treated with cold demonstrated a significant decrease in circumferential measurement at the mid-patellar level and additionally noted some subjective diminution in pain.

Given the lack of definitive benefit of heat to cold or vice versa, the choice of modality should be determined by patient preference and the presence of acute or chronic inflammation.

Application

Cold agents transfer energy either by conduction or evaporation. Conduction occurs when the cold application directly contacts the body surface and these agents include ice/cold packs, ice massage, and immersion in cold water or slush baths. Vapocoolant sprays achieve cooling by evaporation. No cold modality has been demonstrated to be superior over another and investigators have tended to compare the effects of heat to cold rather than one form of cold application to another.

The choice of cold agent should depend on availability, the area to be treated, and patient reaction. Ice massage and vapocoolant sprays are most effective over a small area such as a bursa or trigger point while cold/slush baths are more appropriate for larger, more irregular surfaces. Cold packs and iced towels provide effective cooling when wrapped around joints such as the knees, or when laid over a muscle. Cold compression units maintain a constant cooling temperature and intermittently apply pressure through a sleeve placed over an extremity. Cold may be easily applied in the home setting by commercial cold packs, plastic bags filled with ice cubes, towels soaked in crushed ice, or commercially packaged bags of frozen vegetables such as peas.

The length of cold application varies from a few seconds to 30 minutes, depending on the agent and the part being treated (See Table 6-1 for information on the application of individual cold modalities.)

Precautions

The initial response to a cold application is a sensation of pain, succeeded by numbness. The application should be discontinued if the patient complains of severe pain or discomfort.

Cryotherapy should not be used on patients with Raynaud's phenomenon or other vascular pathology. Other conditions in which cold should be avoided include cryoglobulinemia or paroxysmal cold hemoglobinurias.[53,54] Cold applications should be avoided or increased padding should be used when the application would be over bony prominances or subcutaneous nerves such as the ulnar groove or fibular head. The patient's skin should be closely monitored during treatment and observed for excessive redness or cold urticaria.

HYDROTHERAPY

As early as 4,000 BC Sanskrit writings recorded the healing properties of water and in the third century BC Hippocrates advocated both hot and cold water treatments.[55,56] The Greeks and Romans used water for recreational as well as curative purposes and through succeeding centuries baths continued to be an accepted treatment for a large variety of diseases and conditions. In recent decades the introduction of mechanically controlled agitation added yet another dimension to hydrotherapy, and the current proliferation of hot tubs and spas attests to its continuing popularity for the relief of musculoskeletal aches and pains.

Physical and Mechanical Principles

Hydrotherapy utilizes several principles of physics.[57,58] Among them are: (1) specific gravity, (2) buoyancy, (3) moment of force, and (4) movement through water.

The *specific gravity* of a substance equals the ratio of the weight of that substance to the weight of an equal volume of water. The relative density of water is 1 and the average specific gravity of a body with air in the lungs is estimated to 0.974. Therefore most people will float, or nearly float.

Archimedes' principle of buoyancy states that when a body is fully or partially immersed in a fluid at rest it experiences an upward thrust equal to the weight of the displaced fluid. Buoyancy is a force and can provide either assistance or resistance to movements through water.

The *moment of force* is the turning effect of a force about a fixed point. For a body in water the force is buoyancy and the point is a human joint. As the limb approaches the water surface the turning effect increases, and conversely, decreases as the limb moves deeper into the water. Adding a float or lengthening the lever arm augments the turning affect. The practical importance of this is that buoyancy will assist upward movement towards the water surface and resist movement away from it. Buoyancy and gravity usually balance each other when a limb moves gently in the horizontal plane. Buoyancy can therefore assist, resist, and support movement.

The *flow of a liquid* may be either streamlined or turbulent. Internal friction, or viscosity, increases in turbulent water, making movement through it more difficult. This principle may be used to provide resistance to exercise. Streamlining a body part will facilitate movement.

Water pumps, or turbines, create the mechanical effects of hydrotherapy. The addition of agitation to the water has not been shown to have a significant effect on blood flow and its precise effect on other body tissues has yet to be determined.[59] Nevertheless it seems to aid in the relief of pain, stiffness, and muscle spasm. Walsh has speculated that the agitation acts as a counter-irritant or stimulus to large sensory afferents to block pain input.[60] The sedative and analgesic effect may result from the mechanical stimulation of the skin receptors.

Physiologic Effects

The water's temperature determines the physiologic effects of hydrotherapy. The effects of either hot or cold water will be the same as those covered in the sections on heat and cold. However, they will be more generalized, as a larger body surface is usually immersed in water. Systemic effects occur if a significant portion of the body is submerged for a sufficient length of time.[61] In general, total body cold applications decrease heart rate, increase cardiac muscle tone, and raise blood pressure. Immersion in warm water increases the heart rate, respiratory rate, superficial circulation, and the general metabolic rate. The body temperature usually rises as well.

Indications

Hydrotherapy has been advocated for innumerable conditions including musculoskeletal trauma and fracture,[62,63] neurologic diseases and conditions,[63,64] and wound care and debridement.[65] Pool therapy is often used for specific patient populations such as the elderly.[66,67] For many years it has been a popular choice for physical conditioning.[68,69]

Historically, arthritis and rheumatic conditions have been among the most common indications for hydrotherapy although few controlled studies have been conducted to determine efficacy.[70–72] Baldwin compared pool therapy to an individualized home exercise program for children with juvenile rheumatoid arthritis.[73] Both groups improved although the pool group demonstrated a greater increase in quadriceps strength and the home exercise group showed a greater increase in mobility. Parents and children expressed a preference for the pool program and felt the group socialization experience was especially beneficial. In another study investigators compared the effects on range of motion of a water exercise program to a period of free swimming for children with juvenile rheumatoid arthritis.[74] While the children in both programs benefitted from the activity, most improvement was observed in those participating in the water exercise program.

Although pools have long been a popular choice for physical conditioning exercise, it is only in recent years that programs have been developed and evaluated for arthritis populations. In a long term study Nordemar and associates demonstrated that patients with rheumatoid arthritis could benefit from physical training.[75] Although patients initially began their exercise program on a bicycle ergometer they were allowed to change to another mode of training and many chose swimming as an alternative. More recently Minor and Young evaluated the effects on individuals with either rheumatoid arthritis or osteoarthritis of two physical conditioning exercise protocols, one of which consisted of 12 weeks of exercise in a heated pool.[76,77] Results indicated that the protocol was safe, well accepted, and effective. These investigations hold promise for the use of pool therapy for physical conditioning for individuals with arthritis. However, as with all such programs careful monitoring and appropriate safety precautions must be observed.

The ability of pools to accommodate groups and the resulting interaction and socialization provides an added benefit to pool therapy. Group classes can be developed for specific rheumatic diseases such as ankylosing spondylitis,[78–80] juvenile rheumatoid arthritis,[73,74] and rheumatoid arthritis[76,77] and provide the opportunity for both targeted exercise and socialization. Group adaptive aquatic programs are often available at local community centers and may serve as a valuable adjunct to a therapeutic exercise program. Many YMCAs offer an arthritis aquatic program that was developed in conjunction with the National Arthritis Foundation. However, before referring a patient to a community program the therapist should be thoroughly familiar with the facility, the qualifications of the instructor, and the specific program.

Aquatic Exercise

One of the primary advantages of hydrotherapy for individuals with arthritis lies in the benefits derived from the decreased stress on joints and the sensation of weightlessness produced by buoyancy. Ambulation that normally is painful and difficult may be performed in a pool with much greater ease due to the decreased weight bearing.

Exercises to be performed in a whirlpool, Hubbard tank, and especially a pool, should be carefully designed to take advantage of the principles of aquatics. Buoyancy acts in the opposite direction of gravity and exercise programs that may be appropriate out of the water could be inappropriate in water.

Manuals and books describing specific exercises and programs are available.[81,82] Additionally, techniques[83] utilizing proprioceptive neuromuscular facilitation patterns have been developed for aquatics and inexpensive quantitative approaches[84] to measuring and applying resistance under water have been described. Therapists who have pool facilities available or who prescribe home or community pool exercise programs should familiarize themselves with the scope and diversity of exercises possible in the aquatic setting.

Application

Hydrotherapy transmits energy by conduction and includes any agent or device in which a body or a body part may be immersed in water. Whirlpools, lowboys, and Hubbard tanks are found in most physical therapy departments. Therapeutic pools are much less common but offer innumerable advantages in the treatment of individuals with arthritis. Methods through which hydrotherapy may be applied in the home or community setting include bathtubs, swimming pools, spas, or hot tubs. Showers may be more feasible for those individuals with limited mobility that precludes entering a bathtub. Hydrotherapy is not as portable as some modalities but warm water soaks of the feet or hands may be easily achieved.

Although all methods may use either hot or cold water, warm to hot is certainly most common. Contrast baths alternate hot with cold and have been recommended for the relief of morning stiffness and the reduction of swelling.[85,86] With the exception of contrast baths, the length of applications depends to a great extent on the temperature of the water and the amount of the body submerged. (See Table 6-1 for information on the application of the various forms of hydrotherapy.)

Precautions

Similar precautions for hot and cold hydrotherapy should be observed as for other types of heat and cold applications. Patients should be instructed on the correct temperature and length of time for home baths, showers, and pool activities. Patients exercising in very warm pools are especially vulnerable to fatigue. Accessibility can be difficult and the therapist should assess the patients' ability to etner bathtubs, showers, and pools at home.

Other aspects of hydrotherapy require careful evaluation and monitoring. Individuals receiving pool therapy should be evaluated for water safety and should not be left unattended during treatment. Patients with arthritis, who are normally water safe, may experience balance and coordination problems due to pain, weakness, and limited joint mobility. Incontinence, open wounds, skin infections, and contagious rashes are clearly contraindicated in pool therapy. Other contraindications include fever, cardiac failure, and severely diminished vital capacity. Although it has been suggested that individuals with ankylosing spondylitis should not participate in pool therapy if they have a diminished vital capacity, this has not been demonstrated to be true.[80]

Since hydrotherapy often includes exercise, therapists should observe precautions similar to those for exercising out of the water while still taking into consideration that joint stress is considerably reduced. This advantage makes hydrotherapy, especially pool therapy, particularly valuable in the treatment of patients with arthritis.

TRANSCUTANEOUS ELECTRICAL NERVE STIMULATION

Scientists have realized for centuries that the human body is an electrical phenomenon and have attempted to alter its function through the use of electricity. Hippocrates and the early Egyptians experimented with natural forms of electricity to modify pain.[87] Crude devices capable of generating galvanic current were developed over two centuries ago but, although extensively used for pain control, electricity was generally viewed as a largely unscientific modality employed by individuals on the health care fringe. The popularity of electricity waxed and waned until the mid 1960s when Melszak and Wall postulated their gate control theory of pain.[88] Clinical interest reawakened as their work provided an acceptable scientific basis for electrical neuromodulation of pain.

Neurophysiologic Mode of Action

The gate theory proposes that a "gate" for pain exists in the substantia gelatinosa of the posterior spinal horns. Small diameter A-delta and C fibers carry impulses generated by noxious painful stimuli to the spinal cord. Selective stimulation of large diameter myelinated cutaneous afferent nerve fibers block these pain impulses at their synapse, preventing them from reaching higher levels of the central nervous system. Increased activity in the large diameter myelinated fibers closes the gate, while increased activity in the small fibers tends to open the gate.

Although the gate control theory gave impetus to the use of electricity for pain relief and has been proposed as a possible explanation for the transcutaneous electrical nerve stimulation (TENS) mode of action, it cannot account for pain relief in many clinical conditions or for TENS' long-term analgesic effect. More recent investigation suggests that electrical stimulation may release endogenously produced opiates, called endorphins, or enkephalins.[89] However, it has not yet been demonstrated that the application of TENS might initiate the release of endorphins. As the effect of TENS may be both local and generalized it seems most probable that a number of neurologic mechanisms may be involved.

Indications

TENS was first applied to screen and select patients for surgical implantation of dorsal column stimulators. Clinicians began to use it as a therapeutic device when it became apparent that it alone often produced sufficient pain relief. Since then TENS has been used extensively to alleviate both acute and chronic pain. As it may potentially produce relief during treatment and extend relief following stimulation, it has been employed for a variety of medical and surgical conditions.

The clinical effectiveness of TENS in the management of acute pain, especially postoperative pain, is well documented. Surgical procedures for which significant pain relief was achieved have included laparotomy[90], cholecystectomy,[87] and laminectomy.[91] TENS has also been applied to modify the pain of other acute conditions including muscle sprains and ligamentous strains,[92] acute dental pain,[93] Sudeck's atrophy,[94] and childbirth.[95]

TENS has been used extensively for chronic pain control, most notably for relief of low back pain.[96–98] Investigators also report relief for post-herpetic neuralgia and other painful neuropathies.[99] Objective evaluation of TENS for chronic pain conditions is often complicated by many extenuating factors. Medications, other past and current treatments, and psychological aspects make TENS' efficacy difficult to assess. Etiologies vary extensively and may be unclear or unknown, and assessment tools may be imprecise and not sufficiently objective. Nevertheless, TENS appears to offer relief for individuals with diagnoses and symptom complexes that are associated with chronic pain.

Theoretically TENS should ameliorate joint pain, as C fibers supply the joint synovium, periosteum, and capsule. TENS has been widely applied for the management of musculoskeletal and arthritis pain. Mannheimer et al reported significant relief of wrist pain in 95 percent of their patients with rheumatoid arthritis treated with high intensity TENS.[100] Kumar and Reford applied TENS to the wrists of 20 patients with rheumatoid arthritis and recorded excellent relief in 80 percent of the patients.[89] Abelson et al evaluated the effect of TENS on resting pain and pain while gripping, and improvement was noted in both parameters.[101] Grip strength, measured as power and work done, increased after each treatment but returned to normal between treatments. Other studies also document increased short term, but limited long term relief with TENS.[97]

TENS has been used with limited success for pain secondary to osteoarthritis. Lewis et al reported inconclusive results in a trial of self-administered and placebo TENS for 30 patients with osteoarthritis of the knee.[102] Although 60 percent noted greater than 50 percent pain relief, there was a 43 percent placebo response. Taylor et al evaluated both short and long term response to TENS using actual TENS and a placebo unit.[103] Actual TENS provided more pain relief and most patients claimed the best results were achieved while the unit was operating. Although relief often lasted several hours following treatment, they reported little long-term relief after the test month.

Harvie demonstrated the effectiveness of TENS as an adjunct to rehabilitation.[104] He evaluated TENS for the management of postoperative knee pain on patients with a variety of knee surgical procedures, including total knee replacements. Patients treated with TENS were able to decrease narcotic use and achieve increased quadriceps strength, knee range of motion, and earlier ambulation. Length of hospital stay was decreased.

Other musculoskeletal conditions for which investigators report success include adhesive capulitis[105] and muscle pain associated with muscle spasm and/or tightness.[106] Back pain associated with osteoporosis may also be responsive to TENS.

Quantification of Pain Relief

Precise quantification of pain relief for rheumatic diseases has plagued investigators of TENS. Although relief of acute pain may be easier to assess than chronic pain, the validity of measurement tools is still a major concern. Techniques for evaluating the analgesic effect of TENS vary considerably among studies, often making interpretation of the results difficult. Many investigators have utilized measures of increased loading time or grip strength, although the choice of weight, loading time, and correlation with degree of pain relief varied among individual studies. Mannheimer reported that pain relief measured by weight-loading wrists of patients with rheumatoid arthritis correlated well with patient self-report.[107]

The placebo response must be considered when evaluating the effectiveness of TENS. Several investigators have attempted to assess the level of placebo response for patients with rheumatoid arthritis.[89,101-103] Results ranged from 17 percent[101] to 43 percent,[102] which is similar to the placebo effect noted in studies of analgesic medication. While it is not usually feasible for the clinician to evaluate the placebo response on a patient by patient basis it should be taken into consideration when assessing the results of treatment.

The patient chart should include documentation of changes in pain level. Pain measurement scales should be completed before and following treatment. Therapists should also record changes in pain medication, functional ability, strength, range of motion, and gait. Pain measurement scales should be administered at intervals following treatment to determine whether there has been any long-term relief from TENS.

Application

Clinicians and investigators have employed many methods of application as optimal stimulation characteristics and placement locations have not yet been determined. Relatively few investigators have attempted to compare variations in pulse shape, duration, and intensity, and specific treatment methods are often incompletely described in the literature. Mannheimer evaluated three different frequencies and demonstrated that the analgesic effect of TENS was better with high intensity stimulation.[107] Initially the lowest pulse width setting available on a unit should be selected in order to provide a stimulus of sufficient intensity to large-diameter afferent fibers without stimulating motor fibers and the smaller diameter nocioceptive fibers. The amplitude should be slowly increased until the patient feels a strong tingling at the site of application. Further adjustments of pulse width and amplitude may be necessary in order to elicit the desired sensation or if motor activity occurs.

Investigators have also experimented with a variety of electrode placement sites. Optimal placement for joint pain appears to be directly over the point of pain while placement over appropriate myotomes or scleratomes may be beneficial for muscular pain.[108] Harvie found that for postoperative knee joint pain, placement over the medial and lateral collateral ligaments produced the best results.[104] Remote stimulation has not been studied extensively for rheumatic disease pain, but the results of one study suggests that it may not be effective.[107]

Clinicians should base their choice of setting and electrode placement on their clinical experience and the individual patient's response to treatment. Several trials may be necessary before optimal results are achieved.

Precautions

TENS is notable for the absence of undesirable side effects. Problems most frequently encountered include an adverse reaction of the skin to electricity, the tape, or a conducting medium or aversion to the sensation (paresthesia)

TENS produces. TENS should be used cautiously on patients with sclero-derma, vasculitis, or sensory neuropathic lesions. Potentially serious side ef-fects could include cardiac arrhythmia and interference with cardiac pace-makers, and TENS should not be used on patients with these complications. An unusual case of a dramatic neurovascular response to TENS was docu-mented in a woman with rheumatoid arthritis[109]; no other serious side effects have been reported in individuals with rheumatic diseases. However, patients experiencing significant pain relief from TENS should use their joints cau-tiously and be warned to avoid activities which could unduly stress joints and cause further damage.

More studies must be conducted to definitively establish TENS' clinical effectiveness and determine the optimal parameters of wave-form, setting, and placement. The effect on strength, range of motion, and ambulation, as well as pain control, should be an important thrust of investigation. Nevertheless, TENS is firmly established as an effective, although potentially expensive mo-dality. Therapists should carefully assess the effectiveness of TENS, deter-mining whether another, less expensive, modality might be equally as effective. Cost must be balanced with efficacy when clinicians and patients choose a modality.

TRACTION

Skeletal traction has been used to realign dislocations and reduce fractures since at least the time of Hippocrates.[110] Illustrations of ancient Greek traction apparatus demonstrate design and application principles that, although primi-tive by contemporary standards, are remarkably similar to those of equipment in use today. Traction continues to play a major role in the treatment of frac-tures and other orthopedic conditions and for the past several decades spinal traction has been used to relieve neck and back pain believed to result from nerve root compression.

Mode of Action

The actual mechanism by which traction relieves pain is unknown although it is generally assumed that pain relief is obtained from stretching and separating vertebral structures, reducing pressure on herniating discs, and allowing them to recede. Traction might also stretch the posterior ligaments of the interver-tebral foramen and increase the space available for the nerve root. Studies on normal individuals and cadavers demonstrate that large forces can achieve vertebral separation, especially of the cervical vertebrae.[111-113] It is unclear, however, if this is true in the presence of joint and disc pathology.[114] It is also unclear whether vertebral separation is even necessary for pain relief and if so, how much is required. Whether or not vertebral separation is achieved, the application of passive stretch to tonically contracting paraspinal muscles may induce muscle relaxation and the stimulation of stretch receptors may alter pain perception. Furthermore, the slight separation and stretching of ligamentous and bony structures may allow increased circulation and improved nutrition to compressed structures.[115] However, it is questionable whether traction can provide significant and lasting relief for pain resulting from root impingement, especially if the source of the impingement is unaffected. Continuous lumbar traction does enforce bedrest and is frequently advocated solely for this reason.[114,116,117]

Indications

Traction has been used extensively to relieve the pain associated with degenerative intervertebral disc disease. Evidence of osteoarthritis and disc degeneration can be found in most people over 50 years old, although many are asymptomatic.[110] Correlations have not been found between osteophyte formation and disc degeneration or between radiologic changes and root compression symptoms[118], and symptoms often abate whether or not treatment is instituted. This lack of a direct relationship between pathology and symptomatology complicates the task of determining the clinical effectiveness of traction.

Historically, most studies have explored the issue of vertebral separation rather than treatment efficacy in terms of pain relief. Those investigations which did look at efficacy varied greatly in design, application, and measurement with no definitive conclusions. Furthermore, investigators usually included several treatment modalities (e.g., heat and massage), so that it is difficult to determine whether traction alone effected the improvement. In a study of 61 patients with cervical disc syndrome, Martin and Corbin documented improvement in 67.2 percent on a regimen of heat, massage, and traction.[119] Steinberg and Mason randomly assigned patients with cervical pain attributable to degenerative disease to one of three treatment groups:[120] (1) heat, massage, and traction; (2) neck and shoulder girdle exercises; and (3) cervical collar. At the end of 1 month the results for all groups were similar, with a 73 percent overall improvement rate. Shenkin treated 27 patients who were felt to be surgical candidates for root compression symptoms with cervical traction.[121] Sixteen recovered sufficiently so as to not require surgery. In a controlled study arranged by the British Association of Physical Medicine, 466 patients with root compression symptomatology were randomly assigned to one of five treatment groups.[122] Cervical traction was compared to head and neck positioning simulating traction, posture instruction and a soft collar, placebo medication, and untuned short wave diathermy. Results indicated that while the majority of all patients exhibited decreased pain and increased range of motion and function, there was not a statistically significant difference between groups. Pain relief achieved with traction was not significantly better than that achieved with simple positioning without traction.

There are even fewer studies on intermittent lumbar traction for osteoarthritic changes. Masturzo reported that eight out of ten patients with definite osteoarthritic changes did not improve with lumbar traction.[123] The results of other studies on traction for disc degeneration[124] and ruptured intervertebral discs[125] are generally more favorable with over 50 percent improvement noted.[125] Continuous lumbar traction is frequently used for the management of discogenic pain although the goals of treatment are usually immobilization rather than vertebral separation.

Application

Cervical Traction

Most research into traction has explored the intriguing question of whether it produces sufficient vertebral separation to relieve compressed or impinged structures. If so, how much force, applied for how long, in what position, and at what angle, is necessary? Many of these issues are still unresolved although less so for cervical traction. Halter placement, angle of rope pull, tractive force, and duration of traction are interrelated and the results of at least one study indicates a definite relationship between the amount of vertebral body separation, amount of tractive force, and angle of rope pull.[111] Judovich and Nobel determined that at least 30 to 35 pounds was necessary to achieve vertebral separation.[112] Colachis and Strohm studied the effect of 30 and 50 pounds of traction at several angles of pull.[111] They found that a tractive force of 30 pounds for 7 seconds could separate the cervical vertebrae posteriorly. Anteriorly, the changes were less specific and were related more to the angle of pull than to the tractive force.

The duration of time necessary to achieve separation has also preoccupied investigators. Colachis and Strohm studied the amount of separation achieved with a tractive force of 30 pounds applied for 25 minutes of intermittent traction.[126] Results indicated that the amount of separation increased as the period of application increased with a maximum separation at 25 minutes. Intervals of pull of 7, 30, or 60 seconds did not produce any difference in separation and 20 minutes after separation a statistically significant amount of anterior separation was still present although no posterior separation remained.

Currently, the clinical application of cervical traction for degenerative disc disease and root compression symptoms varies greatly as the optimal force, position, duration, and angle of pull have yet to be determined. Forces of 15 to 30 pounds[114,127] have been advocated although clinical investigations have utilized higher forces.[119,121] The clinician should start with a relatively low weight sufficient to counterbalance the weight of the head and progress to 25 to 30 pounds until maximum pain relief is achieved. Patient comfort should be the major consideration during treatment as the ability to tolerate tractive forces will vary among individuals. Intermittent traction can be applied in either the supine or sitting position. Most commonly it is given with the patient seated, although once again patient comfort should be the primary concern. Patients are usually positioned in cervical flexion and 24° is generally assumed to provide optimal separation of the vertebral interspaces.[126,128]

Twenty to 30 minutes is usually considered the maximum time for total duration of treatment but there is no consensus on the amount of time that pull should alternate with rest for intermittent traction, or the amount of pull time necessary for continuous traction. Due to the versatility of timing and amount of force available from an intermittent traction machine, complex regimens have been advanced. Therapists should choose the pull-rest interval cycle with which they have the best empirical success and which affords the patient the most relief.

Cervical traction may be effectively reproduced in the home setting. Commercial traction units which usually utilize over-the-door placement are readily available. Patients should face the door with their head positioned in slight flexion and the halter should pull equally under the mandible and the occiput, avoiding stress on potentially painful temporomandibular joints. The comprehensive home program should include instructions for total treatment time, amount of tractive force, and pull-rest cycles. Several methods for achieving an effective tractive force include the use of weights as a counterbalance or the weight of a relaxed, sagging upper body.[129]

Lumbar Traction

The question of whether lumbar traction produces vertebral separation and how much is required to do so is more difficult to answer than it is for cervical traction. Estimates on the amount necessary have varied from 40 to 800 pounds (depending on the specific joint and the mechanical resistance of the apparatus).[111] Judavich determined that an amount equal to approximately one fourth of the total body weight is required to overcome surface resistance.[112] Twenty-five to 50 percent is commonly assumed to be necessary when traction is applied horizontally on a split traction table.[114] Unquestionably a large force is necessary to achieve even a satisfactory stretch of soft tissue structures. Low forces of 20 pounds or less should be applied continuously as the only advantage to be gained is the enforced bed rest and immobilization. Most commonly, 50 to 80 or 100 pounds of force are used for intermittent traction, depending on the size of the patient and whether a friction-free, split traction table is used.

A study to determine the influence of hip position on vertebral separation during intermittent traction indicated that maximum posterior vertebral separation at rest occurred with subjects positioned in 90° hip flexion.[130] Traction further increased the posterior intervertebral separation. When treated with intermittent lumbar traction, patients should be positioned with their hips in flexion and thoracic and lumbar corsets should both be used to anchor them.

Alternative methods of applying lumbar traction such as inverted positioning[131] and gravitational lumbar traction[132] utilize body weight and/or gravity as the tractive force. Because they do not require complicated machinery these methods may be reproduced at home. Nevertheless, no controlled studies have been conducted to evaluate the efficacy much less the superiority of these methods to the more conventional method of application.

Precautions

Contraindications include the presence of malignancy, acute trauma, osteoporosis, spinal infections, and evidence of cord compression.[110] Traction should be discontinued in patients who experience increased pain during treatment. Although intermittent cervical traction has been suggested for the pain resulting from rheumatoid arthritis of the cervical spine[133] it will not achieve reduction of subluxations or correct associated myelopathies and should be used cautiously, if at all. It is contraindicated in the presence of active synovitis.

Although the effectiveness of traction is essentially supported by anecdotal evidence, cervical traction appears to offer some benefit to the individual with obvious radiculopathy associated with disc disease. The benefits of lumbar traction lie primarily in the artificially imposed immobilization. Until controlled studies using sophisticated research designs and measurement tools are conducted, the effectiveness of traction as an effective modality for the relief of pain associated with root compression remains in doubt.

BIOFEEDBACK

Although the concept of mind over matter is scarcely new, the development and use of biofeedback in recent decades makes it the most recent modality. In essence, biofeedback provides information to the subject about his or her physiologic functions. Electronic equipment monitors specific body processes such as skin temperature, blood pressure, heart rate, and muscle contractions. Bodily processes produce signals which are displayed for the subject. With training, subjects can learn to modify and control these processes, thus gaining a form of voluntary control over their body's behavior. Depending upon their specific problem an individual can utilize the information received through biofeedback and learn how to modify the physiologic processes that aggravate the condition.

Biofeedback has been used for a wide variety of conditions including muscle spasticity, tension headaches, and gait deviations.[134] In the rheumatic diseases biofeedback has primarily been employed in the treatment of vasoconstrictive syndromes and as a pain control measure.[135-137] Investigators have used biofeedback to teach relaxation techniques and modify physiologic reactions to stresses which can increase arthritis pain.[138] Although not yet in common use for arthritis and other rheumatic conditions, biofeedback holds promise as an alternative approach for the relief of chronic pain. Qualified therapists with specialized training in the use of the equipment and procedures should explore the uses of biofeedback in the treatment of their patients with arthritis.

REFERENCES

Heat

1. Licht S: History of therapeutic heat. In Licht S (ed): Therapeutic Heat and Cold. E. Licht, New Haven, 1965
2. Erlich G: Treatment of rheumatoid arthritis. JAMA 228:94, 1974
3. Smyth CJ: Therapy of rheumatoid arthritis: A pyramidal plan. Postgrad Med 51:31, 1972
4. Ward AWM, Williams BT, Dixon RA: Physiotherapy: its prescription and implementation for orthopaedic outpatients. Rheumatol Rehabil 17:14, 1978
5. In Lehman JF (ed): Therapeutic Heat and Cold. Williams & Wilkins, Baltimore, 1982
6. Fountain FP, Gersten JW, Sengir O: Decrease in muscle spasm produced by ultrasound, hot packs, and infrared radiation. Arch Phys Med Rehabil 41:293, 1960
7. Lehman JF, Masock A, Warren G, Koblanski J: Effect of therapeutic temperatures on tendon extensibility. Arch Phys Med Rehabil 51:481, 1970
8. Lehman JF, Brunner GD, Stow RW: Pain threshold measurements after therapeutic application of ultrasound, microwave and infrared. Arch Phys Med Rehabil 39:560, 1958
9. Downey JA: Physiological effects of heat and cold. Phys Ther 44:713, 1964
10. Lehman JF, Gerald WG, Seham SM: Therapeutic heat and cold. Clin Orthop 99:207, 1974
11. Wright V, Johns RJ: Physical factors concerned with the stiffness of normal and diseased joints. Bull Johns Hopkins Hosp 106:215, 1960
12. Tepperman PS, Devlin M: Therapeutic heat and cold. A practitioner's guide. Postgrad Med 73:69, 1983
13. Hollander JL, Horvath SM: Influence of physical therapy procedures on intra-articular temperatures of normal and arthritic subjects. Am J Med Sci 218:543, 1949
14. Horvath SM, Hollander JL: Intra-articular temperature as a measure of joint reaction. J Clin Invest 28:469, 1949
15. Harris ED Jr, McCroskery JA: Influence of temperature and fibril stability on degradation of cartilage collagen by rheumatoid synovial collagenase. N Engl J Med 290:1, 1974
16. Freibel A, Fast A: Deep heating of joints: A reconsideration. Arch Physic Med Rehabil 57:513, 1976
17. Abramson DI, Abramson DI, Bell Y, Rejalh H, et al: Changes in blood flow, O_2 uptake and tissue temperatures produced by therapeutic physical agents: I. Effects of ultrasound. Am J Phys Med 39:51, 1960
18. Aldes JH, Jadenson WJ, Grabinski S: A new approach to the treatment of subdeltoid bursitis. Am J Physic Med 33:79, 1954
19. Gersten JW: Effect of ultrasound on tendon extensibility. Am J Phys Med 34:362, 1955
20. Gerber LH: Principles and their application in the rehabilitation of patients with

rheumatic disease. In Kelley WN, Harris ED, Jr, et al (eds): Textbook of Rheumatology. Vol II. WB Saunders Co, Philadelphia, 1981

21. Swezey RL: Essentials of physical management and rehabilitation in arthritis. Semin Arthritis Rheum 3:349, 1974
22. Flax HJ: Ultrasound treatment of peritendinitis. Calcarea of the shoulder. Am J Physic Med 43:117, 1964
23. Gallagher LA, Eshleman JK, Schumacher HR: A controlled study of the effects of paraffin baths on the rheumatoid hand. Unpublished abstract presented at 1980 ARA/AHPA Annual Scientific Meeting, 1980
24. Harris R, Millard JP: Paraffin wax baths in the treatment of rheumatoid arthritis. Ann Rheum Dis 14:278, 1955
25. Cordray YM, Krusen EM Jr.: Use of hydrocollator packs in the treatment of neck and shoulder pains. Arch Physic Med Rehabil 40:105, 1959
26. Lee PN, Lee M, Hag AM, Longton EB, Wright V: Periarthritis of the shoulder. Trial of treatments investigated by multivariate analysis. Ann Rheum Dis 33:116, 1974
27. Weiss JJ, Thompson GR, Doust V, Burgener F: Rotator cuff tears in rheumatoid arthritis. Arch Intern Med 135:521, 1975
28. Erdman II WJ, Stoner, EK: Comparative heating effects of moistaire and hydrocollator hot packs. Arch Physic Med Rehabil 37:71, 1956
29. Abramson D, Tuck S, Lee L, Richardson G, Levin M, Buso E: Comparison of wet and dry heat in raising the temperature of tissues. Arch Physic Med Rehabil 48:654, 1967
30. Abramson D, Tuck S, Luke S, Cesar D: Effect of paraffin bath and hot fomentations on local tissue temperatures. Arch Physic Med Rehabil 45:87, 1964
31. Brewer E: Reduction of morning stiffness and/or pain using a sleeping bag. Pediatrics 56:621, 1975

Cryotherapy

32. Drez D, Faust D, Evans P: Cryotherapy and nerve palsy. Am J Sports Med 9:256, 1981
33. Michlovitz SL: Cryotherapy: The use of cold as a therapeutic agent. p. 78. In Michlovitz SL (ed): Thermal Agents in Rehabilitation. FA Davis, Philadelphia, 1986
34. Fox RH: Local cooling in man. Br Med Bull 17:14, 1961
35. Lewis T: Observations on some normal and injurious effects of cold upon the skin and underlying tissues. Br Med J 2:795, 1941
36. Tepperman PS, Devlin M: Therapeutic heat and cold: A practitioner's guide. Postgrad Med 73:69, 1983
37. Clarke RSJ, Hellon RF, Lind AR: The duration of sustained contractions of the human forearm at different muscle temperatures. J Physiol 143:454, 1958
38. Levine MG, Kabat H, Knott M, et al: Relaxation of spasticity by physiological techniques. Arch Physic Med Rehabil 35:214, 1954
39. DonTigny RL and Sheldon KW: Simultaneous use of heat and cold in treatment of muscle spasm. Arch Phys Med Rehabil 43:235, 1962
40. Baggie Therapy: Simple pain relief for arthritic knees. JAMA 246:317, 1981

41. Utsinger PD, Bonner F, and Hogan N: Efficacy of cryotherapy and thermotherapy in the management of rheumatoid arthritis pain: Evidence for endorphin effect (abstr). Arthritis Rheum 25:S113, 1982
42. Bierman W: Therapeutic Use of Cold. JAMA 157:1189, 1955
43. Grant, AE: Massage with ice (cryokinetics) in the treatment of painful conditions of the musculoskeletal system. Arch Physic Med Rehabil 45:233, 1964
44. Rembe, EC: use of cryotherapy on the post-surgical rheumatoid hand. Phys Ther 50:19, 1970
45. Michlovitz, SL: Cryotherapy: The use of cold as a therapeutic agent. p. 89. In Michlovitz, SL (ed): Thermal Agents in Rehabilitation. FA Davis, Philadelphia, 1986
46. Lane LE: Localized hypothermia for the relief of pain in musculoskeletal injuries. Phys Ther 51:182, 1971
47. Swezey RL: Essentials of physical management and rehabilitation in arthritis. Semin Arthritis Rheum 3:349, 1974
48. Heat and cold as analgesics. Med Lett Drugs Ther 12:3, Jan 9, 1970
49. Hogan NC, Lockard JC, Utsinger PD: Cryotherapy in the management of intractable knee pain in patients with rheumatoid arthritis. (Abst.) ARA/AHPA Annual Scientific Meeting. June, 1981
50. Kirk JA, Kersley GD: Heat and cold in the physical treatment of rheumatoid arthritis of the knee—A controlled clinical trial. Ann Phys Med 9:270, 1968
51. Clarke GR, Willis LA, Stenner L, Nichols PJR: Evaluation of physiotherapy in the treatment of osteoarthritis of the knee. Rheumatol Rehabil 13:190, 1974
52. Hecht PJ, Bachmann S, Booth RE, Rothman RH: Effects of thermal therapy on rehabilitation after total knee arthroplasty. Clin Orthop 178:198, 1983
53. Simpsen CF: Heat, cold or both? Amer J Nurs Feb. 1983, 270–273
54. Bardwick PA, Swezey RL: Physical modalities for treating the foot affected by connective tissue diseases. Foot Ankle 3:41, 1982

Hydrotherapy

55. Blumenthal D: Taking a bath. New York Times Nov. 25, 1984, p. 114
56. Duffield MH: Introduction. In Skinner AT, Thomson AM (eds): Duffield's Exercise in Water. 3rd ed. Balliere Tindall, London, 1983
57. Duffield MH: p. 4. In Skinner AT, Thomson AM (eds): Duffield's Exercise in Water 3rd ed. Balliere Tindall, London, 1983
58. Stewart JB: Exercises in water. p. 291. In Licht S (ed): Therapeutic Exercise. E. Licht, New Haven, 1961
59. Cohen A, Martin G, Wakim K: The effect of whirlpool bath with and without agitation on the circulation in normal and diseased extremities. Arch Phys Med Rehabil 30:212, 1949
60. Walsh M: Hydrotherapy: The use of water as a therapeutic agent. p. 123. In Michlovitz S (ed); Thermal Agents in Rehabilitation. FA Davis, Philadelphia, 1986
61. Walsh M: Hydrotherapy: The use of water as a therapeutic agent. p. 122. In Michlovitz S (ed) Thermal Agents in Rehabilitation. FA Davis, Philadelphia, 1986
62. Lapidus PW, Guidotti FP: Immediate mobilization and swimming pool exercises in some fractures of foot and ankle bones. Clin Orthop 56:197, 1968
63. Chespesvik MW: Underwater exercises in neurologic lesions. In Licht S (ed) Medical Hydrology. E Licht, New Haven, 1963

64. Gehlsen GM, Grigsby JA, Winant DM: Effects of an aquatic fitness program on the muscular strength of patients with multiple sclerosis. Phys Ther 64:653, 1984

65. Walsh M: Hydrotherapy: The use of water as a therapeutic agent. p. 122. In Michlovitz, S (ed) Thermal Agents in Rehabilitation. FA Davis, Philadelphia, 1986

66. Kimble D: A case study in adaptive-aquatics for the geriatric population. Clinic Manag Phys Ther 6:8, 1986

67. Kacavas JJ, Morrison D, Hurley M: The use of aqua therapy with geriatric patients. Am Correc Ther J 31:52, 1977

68. Leach RE: Rx Exercise: Effects and side effects. Hosp Pract Jan:72A, 1981

69. Blocker WP: Physical activities. Postgrad Med 60:56, 1976

70. Daggett R, Gillespie A: Pool therapy in the treatment of rheumatoid arthritis. In Lamont Havers RW, Hislop HJ (eds): Arthritis and Related Disorders American Physical Therapy Association, 1965

71. Swezey RL: Arthritis: Rational Therapy and Rehabilitation. WB Saunders, Philadelphia 1978

72. Wickersham BA: Hydrotherapy. p. 131. In Gall EP Riggs. GD (eds): Rheumatic Diseases: Rehabilitation and Management. Butterworth (Publishers), London, 1984

73. Baldwin J: Pool therapy compared with individual home exercise therapy for juvenile rheumatoid arthritic patients. Physiotherapy 58:230, 1972

74. Vostrejs M, Hollister JR: The effectiveness of an aquanastics program. Arthritis Rheum 28:S150, 1985

75. Nordemar R, Erblom B, Zachrisson L, Londquist K: Physical training in rheumatoid arthritis: A controlled long term study I. Scand J Rheumatol 10:17, 1981

76. Minor MA, Hewett JE, Kay DR: Monitoring for harmful effects of physical conditioning exercise (PGE) with arthritis patients. Arthritis Rheum 29:S144, 1986

77. Young AG, Minor MA: Physical conditioning exercise (PCE) for arthritis patients: Description of method. Arthritis Rheum 29:S144, 1986

78. Harrison RA: Tolerance of pool therapy by ankylosing spondylitis patients with low vital capacities. Physiotherapy 67:296. 1981

79. Harrison RA, Dixon ASJ: Group treatment for ankylosing spondylitis. Rehabilitation, British Health Care and Technology, 1975

80. Mack M. Ankylosing spondylitis fitness course: An education and exercise review program. Arthritis Rheum 30:559, 1987

81. Duffield MH: Skinner AT, Thomson AM, (eds): Duffield's Exercise in Water. 3rd ed. Balliere Tindall, London, 1983

82. Bolton E, Goodwin D: Pool Exercises. 4th ed. Churchill Livingstone, Edinburgh, 1974

83. Boyle AM: The Bad Ragaz Ring Method. Physiotherapy 67:265, 1981

84. Harrison RA: A quantitative approach to strengthening exercises in the hydrotherapy pool. Physiotherapy 66:60, 1980

85. Schuitt A: Physical Medicine and rehabilitation in the elderly arthritis patient. J Am Geriatr Soc 25:76, 1977

86. Bardwick PA, Swezey RL: Physical modalities for treating the foot affected by connective tissue diseases. Foot Ankle 3:41, 1982

Transcutaneous Electrical Nerve Stimulation

87. Rosenberg M, Curtis L, Bourke DL: Transcutaneous electrical nerve stimulation for the relief of postoperative pain. Pain 5:129, 1978
88. Melzack R, Wall PD: Pain mechanisms: A new theory. Science 150:971, 1975
89. Kumar N, Redford SB: Transcutaneous nerve stimulation in rheumatoid arthritis. Arch Phys Med Rehabil 63:595, 1982
90. Schomburg FL, Carter-Baker SA: Transcutaneous electrical nerve stimulation for post-laparotomy pain. Phys Ther 63:188, 1983
91. Schuster GD, Infante MC: Pain relief after low back surgery: The efficacy of TENS. Pain 8:299, 1980
92. Roeser WM, Weeks LW, Venus R, et al: The use of transcutaneous nerve stimulation for pain control in athletic medicine. A preliminary report. Amer J Sports Med 4:210, 1976
93. Hansson P, Ekblom A: TENS as compared to placebo TENS for relief of acute orofacial pain. Pain 15:157, 1983
94. Bodenheim R, Bennett JH: Reversal of a Sudeck's atrophy by the adjunctive use of transcutaneous electrical nerve stimulation: A case report. Phys Ther 63:1287, 1983
95. Augustinsson LE, Bohlin P, Bundsen P, et al.: Pain relief during delivery by transcutaneous electrical nerve stimulation. Pain 4:59, 1977
96. Melzack P, Vetere P, Finch L: Transcutaneous electrical nerve stimulation for low back pain: A comparison of TENS and massage for pain and range of motion. Phys Ther 63:489, 1983
97. Melzack R: Prolonged relief of pain by brief intense transcutaneous somatic stimulation. Pain 1:357, 1975
98. Loeser JD, Black RG, Christman A: Relief of pain by transcutaneous stimulation. J Neurosurg 42:308, 1975
99. Wolf SL, Gersh MR, Rao VR: Examination of electrode placements and stimulating parameters in treating chronic pain with conventional transcutaneous electrical nerve stimulation. Pain 11:37, 1981
100. Mannheimer C, Lund S, Carlsson CA: The effect of transcutaneous electrical nerve stimulation on joint pain in patients with rheumatoid arthritis. Scand J Rheumatol 7:13, 1978
101. Abelson K, Langley GB, Sheppeard H, et al: Transcutaneous electrical nerve stimulation in rheumatoid arthritis. NZ Med J 96:156, 1983
102. Lewis D, Lewis B, Sturrock RD: Transcutaneous electrical nerve stimulation in osteoarthrosis: a therapeutic alternative? Ann Rheum Dis 43:47, 1984
103. Taylor P, Hallett M, Flaherty L. Treatment of Osteoearthritis of the knee with TENS. Pain 11:233, 1981
104. Harvie KW: A major advance in the control of post-operative knee pain. Orthopedics 2:129, 1979
105. Bardwick PA, Swezey RL: Physical therapies in arthritis: which to choose, when to use, how not to abuse. Postgrad Med 72:223, 1982
106. Lampe GN: Introduction to the use of transcutaneous electrical nerve stimulation devices. Phys Ther 58:1450, 1978
107. Mannheimer C, Carlsson CA: The analgesic effect of transcutaneous electrical nerve stimulation in patients with rheumatoid arthritis: A comparative study of different pulse patterns. Pain 6:329, 1979

108. Mannheimer JS: Electrode placements for transcutaneous electrical nerve stimulation. Phys Ther 58:1455, 1978
109. Griffin JW, McClure M: Adverse reactions to transcutaneous electrical nerve stimulation in a patient with rheumatoid arthritis. Phys Ther 61:354, 1981

Traction

110. Licht S: Massage, Manipulation and Traction. E. Licht, New Haven, 1960
111. Colachis SC, Strohn BR: A study of tractive forces and angle of pull on vertebral interspaces in the cervical spine. Arch Phys Med Rehabil 46:820, 1965
112. Judovich B, Nobel GR: Traction Therapy. A study of resistive forces. Amer J Surg 93:108, 1957
113. Harris R: Traction. p. 223. In Licht S (ed): Massage, Manipulation and Traction. E. Licht, New Haven, 1960
114. Swezey RL: Arthritis: Rational Therapy and Rehabilitation. WB Saunders, Philadelphia, 1977
115. Swezey RL: Manual mobilization and traction. p. 190. In Riggs GK, Gall EP (eds): Rheumatic Diseases: Rehabilitation and Management. Butterworth (Publishers), Boston, 1984
116. McQuillan WM: Conservative management of osteoarthritis of the hip. Ann Clin Res 5:49, 1973
117. Oudenhoven RC: Gravitational lumbar traction. Arch Phys Med Rehabil 59:510, 1978
118. Verbiest, H: The management of cervical spondylosis. Clinic Neurosurg 20:262, 1973
119. Martin GM, Corbin KB: An evaluation of conservative treatment for patients with cervical disc syndrome. Arch Physic Med Rehabil 35:87, 1954
120. Steinberg VL, Mason RM: Cervical spondylosis; Pilot therapeutic trial. Ann Phys Med 5:37, 1959
121. Shenkin HA: Motorized intermittent cervical traction for treatment of herniated cervical discs. JAMA 156:1067, 1954
122. British Association of Physical Medicine: Pain in the neck and arm: A multicentre trial of the effects of physiotherapy. Br Med J 1:253, 1966
123. Masturzo A: Vertebral traction for sciatica. Rheumatism 11:62, 1955
124. Lehman JF, Brunner GD: A device for the application of heavy lumbar traction; its mechanical effects. Arch Phys Med Rehabil 39:696, 1958
125. Hood LB, Chrisman D: Intermittent pelvic traction in the treatment of the ruptured intervertebral disc. Phys Ther 48:21, 1968
126. Colachis SC, Strohm BR: Effect of duration of intermittent cervical traction on vertebral separation. Arch of Phys Med Rehabil 47:353, 1966
127. Swezey RL: Essentials of physical management and rehabilitatiion in arthritis. Semin Arthritis Rheum 3:349, 1974
128. Waylonis GW, Tootle D, Denhart C, et al: Home cervical traction: Evaluation of alternate equipment. Arch Phys Med Rehabil 63:388, 1982
129. Laurin CA: Cervical Traction in the home. Can Med Assoc J 94:36, 1966
130. Reilly JP, Gersten JW, Clinkingbeard J: Effect of pelvic-femoral position on vertebral separation produced by lumbar traction. Phys Ther 59:282, 1979
131. Nosse LJ: Inverted spinal traction. Arch Phys Med Rehabil 59:367, 1978

132. Oudenhoven RC: Gravitational lumbar traction. Arch Phys Med Rehabil 59:510, 1978
133. Lipson S: Rheumatoid Arthritis of the cervical spine. Clinic Orthop 182:143, 1984

Biofeedback

134. Wolf SL: Essential considerations in the use of EMG biofeedback. Phys Ther 58:25, 1978
135. Taub E, Stroebel CF: Biofeedback in the treatment of vasoconstrictive syndromes. Biofeedback Self Regul 3:363, 1978
136. Adair JR, Theobald DE: Raynaud's phenomenon: Treatment of a severe case with biofeedback. J Indiana State Med Assoc 21:990, 1978
137. National Institutes of Health: Biofeedback for patients with Raynaud's phenomenon. JAMA 242:509, 1979
138. Achterberg J, McGraw P, Lawlis FG: Rheumatoid arthritis: A study of relaxation and temperature biofeedback training as an adjunctive therapy. Biofeedback Self Regul 6:207, 1981

7 | Gait and Mobility

Phyllis Levine

As the disease processes associated with forms of arthritis become evident in the lower extremity joint structures, inhibition of mobility is quite likely to occur. The altered gait patterns can be explained by considering the specific changes occurring at each joint. A well designed rehabilitation program can and should accommodate these specific physical changes, by teaching the use of appropriate substitution to protect these vulnerable areas. Mobility can then be made as efficient as possible, resulting in a prolonged independent functional status.

Understanding the biomechanics of a normal joint, the pathophysiology of a particular type of arthritis, and the requirements for normal mobility make designing an appropriate program possible. There must be recognition of inadequate capacities, due to specific deformities, to allow for the necessary accommodation. Prolonged ambulation becomes feasible for many persons with arthritis as there are advances in the surgical techniques of joint repair and replacement and the technological qualities of orthotics.

In a global sense, the primary goal of rehabilitation is to restore and/or maintain stability within the range of mobility required for normal activities of daily living at all weight bearing joints. The specific techniques employed to reach this goal will depend on the type of arthritis, the extent of disease and the demands of that person's lifestyle. This chapter will deal primarily with rheumatoid arthritis as it is the complex joint deformities associated with this particular collagen disease that are most commonly and challengingly dealt with in rehabilitation.

BIOMECHANICS OF NORMAL LOWER EXTREMITY JOINTS

The study of mechanics is divided into two parts: kinematics and kinetics. Kinematics is the study of motion of rigid bodies. Kinetics is the study of the forces involved in this motion. As each human joint is a part of an overall complex structure, its mechanics cannot be realistically considered without reviewing the interaction of surrounding joints, and the function of corresponding muscles and ligaments. Muscles provide motion and motion control. Ligaments establish the limits of that motion. Loading forces on the joints are produced by body weight, muscle tension, and external forces. The various lower extremity joints have different capacities to withstand loading forces in static and dynamic situations. Each of the lower extremity joints will be considered independently here and then compositely in an analysis of gait.

The Foot

The biomechanical demands placed on the foot include the extremes of flexibility and stability, to accommodate uneven surfaces in ambulation and provide a rigid lever arm in the late stance phase of gait. Some inherent stability exists in the skeletal architecture of the foot. However, most of the foot's rigidity is attained as a result of external rotation of the leg, which is transmitted to the foot via the subtalar joint. As the hindfoot supinates with heel inversion and lower limb external rotation, the midfoot becomes rigid.[1]

The longitudinal axis of the foot passes between the second and third toes, and is internally rotated 6° to the ankle joint's axis. Available motion about this axis is 0° to 21° of internal rotation and 0° to 9° of external rotation. The axis of rotation of the subtalar joint is oblique. It lies in the transverse plane passing medial to lateral, from distal to proximal at a 23° angle to the foot's midline; the available range of motion there is 4° to 47°. In the horizontal plane, available range of motion is 21° to 69°, and the axis lies at a 41° angle.[1]

Lower extremity rotation will cause calcaneal rotation in the opposite direction. If a failure to rotate occurs at the subtalar joint, transverse rotation will occur at the ankle joint leading to instability there. Thus the subtalar joint acts as a torque transmitter between superior body parts and the ground.[1] It moves in inversion and eversion, with the former range about 0° to 30° and the latter 0° to 10°.

The transverse tarsal joint consists of the talonavicular and the calcaneal cuboid joints. When the hindfoot is supinated (calcaneal inversion) the axes of the transverse tarsal joints are divergent to each other so that restriction of motion occurs. Conversely, with calcaneal eversion, the axes are parallel and free motion occurs. This determines the stability and flexibility of the longitudinal arch of the foot. The navicular articulates with the three cuneiforms and the medial three rays. The cuboid articulates with the lateral two rays. Therefore, with calcaneal inversion the medial border of the foot is elevated and the lateral border depressed, and the opposite occur with heal eversion.

On level ground, weight bearing forces are shared equally between the heel and the forefoot. In the forefoot, the first metatarsal head accepts two times the force of each of the other four metatarsal heads.

The Ankle

The ankle joint consists of the distal tibiofibular joint and the talotibiofibular joint. The latter is more clinically and functionally important. Many ligaments provide stability in this area. The axis of the ankle is just distal to the malleoli. In the transverse plane, the axis of motion is directed laterally and posteriorly while being externally rotated 20° to 30° with respect to the knee axis. In the frontal plane, the axis is lateral and downward. The angle between the ankle axis and the tibia is approximately 80° with a range of 68° to 88°.[1]

Motion occurring at the ankle is 0° to 20° of dorsiflexion and 0° to 50° of plantar flexion. The architectural shape of the talus causes plantar flexion to be accompanied by ankle internal rotation and forefoot varus, while dorsiflexion causes forefoot valgus in ankle external rotation.

The Knee

The knee is usually considered the most complex joint of the body. The knee joint consists of the tibiofemoral and the patellofemoral articulations. The tibiofemoral joint allows motion in the sagittal, transverse, and frontal planes. Most motion occurs in the sagittal plane with 0° to 140° of flexion. External rotation of 0° to 45° and internal rotation of 0° to 30° is seen in the transverse plane at 90° of knee flexion. The frontal plane has only a few degrees of passive abduction and adduction seen with 30° of knee flexion. At the patellofemoral joint, motion occurs simultaneously in the frontal and transverse planes, with greater range of motion in the former.[3] Normal activities of daily living require approximately 117° of active knee flexion.[4] Level ambulation at a self-selected velocity requires approximately 0° to 67° of flexion,[3] a larger range than required of the other lower extremity joints.

The tibiofemoral joint's instant center of motion has a semicircular pathway. External rotation of the tibia on the femur occurs as the tibia slides anteriorly on the femur from flexion to extension. The converse occurs with flexion from extension. This "screw home" mechanism serves to increase stability of the knee at any point in its range. It is this phenomenon that makes this joint not a simple hinge. From extension to full flexion of the knee, analysis of the patellofemoral joint motion shows patellar excursion to be approximately 7 cm in a caudal direction. The patella externally rotates after 90° of flexion. At this point, it only articulates with the medial femoral facet.

The forces that both of these components of the knee joint are subjected to during weight bearing can be several times body weight. The tibial plateau has the primary responsibility for load bearing with the cartilage, menisci, and ligaments sharing in the role.

The Hip

The hip is a highly mobile joint. Fortunately, intrinsic stability is seen here because of the ball and socket configuration. This allows large forces to be borne at the hip joint in the execution of normal activities of daily living. There are three planes of motion between the acetabulum and the femoral head. Normally, 140° of flexion and 15° of extension are seen in the sagittal plane, and 30° of abduction and 20° of adduction in the frontal plane. Rotation in the transverse plane is most freely allowed when accompanied by hip flexion. Normal motion is 90° of external rotation and 70° of internal rotation. The required available hip range of motion to accomplish normal activities of daily living has been estimated at 120° of flexion, 20° of abduction, and 20° of external rotation.[5]

Precise analysis of the instant center of motion is not possible as hip motion simultaneously occurs in three planes. If normal architecture exists, the femoral head will slide tangentially to the surface of the acetabulum. With the architectural changes secondary to rheumatoid arthritis, the joint cartilage is often harmfully compressed or distracted.

The weight bearing forces through the hip joint increase markedly when going from a static state of standing to the dynamic state of ambulation. In single limb stance, 2.5 times body weight is carried at the hip if the gluteus medius is functioning normally to keep the pelvis level.[1] This drops dramatically to 33 percent of body weight in double limb stance as the gluteus medius can be relatively quiet. During gait, the joint reaction force on the femoral head increases from about four times body weight after heel strike to about seven times body weight prior to toe off.[6] Bed rest will not necessarily alleviate joint compression forces as the action of hip flexion and extension, such as needed for the use of a bedpan, brings on forces higher than those needed for crutch or slow ambulation.[7]

When pathology exists at the hip joint, contractures are likely to develop in flexion and external rotation because these are the most restful positions for the hip. Apparent leg length discrepancies occur when this limitation of motion from muscle spasm is present. In either this situation or that of a true leg length inequity due to bone loss, the weight bearing forces will be altered. Secondary degenerative joint disease can be the result of this alteration.

ANALYSIS OF NORMAL GAIT

Gait analysis can be accomplished with varying levels of sophistication. While high technology can provide detailed objective measurements of the various components of gait, for most rehabilitation programs observational analysis provides sufficient information. The walking surface must be level and the patient without shoes. The observer should note the kinematics in each division of gait, looking for compliance or deviation from the known standard patterns. In mid-stance, the position of the subtalar joint must be assessed, as this may affect progression of deformities. If possible, the sole of the shoe should be examined to look for abnormal weight bearing patterns. The speed of ambulation should be self-selected as this will reveal the usual gait pattern for an individual.

The gait cycle is traditionally divided into stance phase and swing phase.

Stance phase is further defined as the contact period being from heel contact of the weight bearing leg to toe off of the contralateral leg; mid-stance from the weight bearing limb's foot flat position to heel lift; and, propulsion from the weight bearing limb's heel lift to toe off. Swing phase begins with a period of acceleration and ends with deceleration. During the beginning and end of stance phase, both lower extremities are in contact with the ground as body weight is transferred from one lower extremity to the other. This is the period of double support and bilaterally, should be of equal duration if gait is symmetrical.

PATHOPHYSIOLOGY OF RHEUMATOID ARTHRITIS IN LOWER EXTREMITY JOINTS

The Forefoot

While 20 percent of patients with rheumatoid arthritis have their initial site of involvement in the foot, 80 percent of those begin in the forefoot.[8-12] The development of hallux valgus, depressed metatarsal heads with distal migration of the plantar fat pad, and hammer and claw toes are the common sequelae (Fig. 7-1).[13]

Since these deformities normally occur early in the disease process, the patients are usually still ambulating. Broadening of the forefoot and separation of the toes occur as a result of peri-articular swelling. Weight bearing on inflammed metatarsophalangeal joints with capsular and ligamentous instability can cause subluxation and eventual dislocation of these joints. If this occurs, the flexor tendons migrate to become functional extensors. The proximal phalanges and plantar fat pad are both drawn distally. This progressive muscle imbalance leads to hammer and claw toe deformities of the four lesser toes and decreased lateral stability of the great toe. Hallux valgus, a lateral migration of the great toe, develops and the important weight bearing capacity of this joint decreases. Decreased stability in ambulation results from the decreased functional length of the foot.[9]

The Hindfoot

Although the hindfoot is less often seen within the foot as an initial site of pathology, results of deformity here can be more debilitating. In a study of 120 patients, 42 percent had some abnormal symptoms of the hindfoot and fully 16 percent found this as their primary cause of disability.[14] Changes developing here are excessive pronation with weight bearing, plantar fasciitis, bursitis, and subplantar spur formation in the heel area. Ambulation clearly aggravates the mechanical stability seen in gait when these hindfoot deformities exist. Midfoot rigidity is directly dependent on hindfoot positioning. If the mid-foot does not lock during weight bearing, the foot is not transformed into a rigid lever

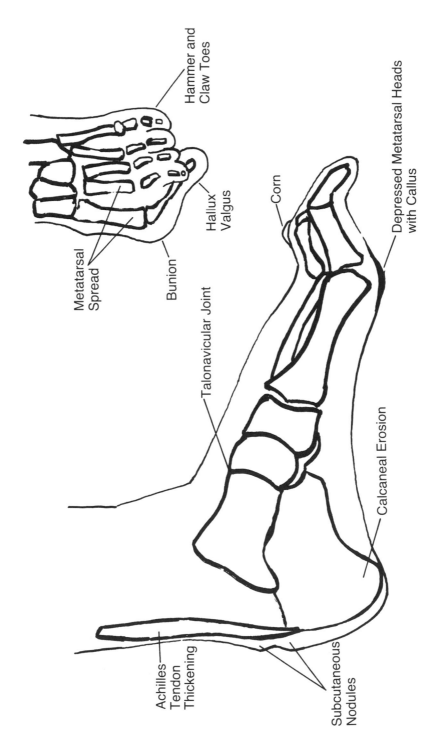

Fig. 7-1. Typical rheumatoid foot deformities.

to allow a safe transfer of weight from the posterior to anterior position. Therefore, excessive pronation in early stance subjects the foot to extreme stress.

The Ankle

The ankle is seldom seen as the site of initial involvement. This is the case with four percent of patients diagnosed as having rheumatoid arthritis.[15] Vidigal et al[15] looked at ankle involvement in 104 patients admitted to a rheumatology unit. Almost 50 percent complained of ankle discomfort, while 12 percent showed radiographic changes at the tibiotalar joint. In the early disease process, tenosynovitis of the posterior tibialis, peroneal and anterior tibialis tendons can occur. Although clinical evidence of this is not often seen, it is commonly noted during surgery. When obvious, a sausage shaped swelling is seen along the course of the tendon.[16] With later rheumatoid arthritic progression, ankle instability develops as there is a loss of cartilage at the articular surface and resultant ligamentous laxity. Erosion of the ligamentous insertions can also occur particularly in the ligament between the tibia and fibula and between these bones and the talus.

With rheumatoid degeneration at the tibiotalar joint, the foot becomes less able to absorb torque from superior body segments. In normal gait, rotation from the leg is imparted to the talus by the grip of the ankle mortise. The subtalar joint then converts this motion into calcaneal rotation in the opposite direction.[2] If the ankle mortise is unable to properly transfer forces to the talus, the subtalar joint cannot respond appropriately.

The Knee

Functional capacity of the knee can be greatly altered by rheumatoid arthritis. Although this joint is a fairly common site for initial pathology, it remains second to the foot in this regard.[12,13] Changes from the disease process can be seen at the tibiofemoral and patellofemoral joint as well as in the surrounding soft tissues. Potter has described the typical rheumatoid arthritic knee deformity as one of flexion, subluxation, valgus, and external rotation.[17] A full knee evaluation should be conducted to assess each of these components. This includes range of motion, muscle strength and length, joint effusion, ligamentous stability, patellar tracking, and bony alignment. Additionally, surrounding joints should be evaluated as prolonged limitation of motion at the knee usually results in hypermobility at these areas. A popliteal cyst may be seen in the popliteal fossa. They are usually asymptomatic unless they rupture.

Any amount of synovitis at the knee alters the instant center of motion of the tibiofemoral joint. This is a precursor to degenerative joint arthritis from abnormal and increased articular compression forces. Extra-articular change is seen as prolonged swelling, and can mechanically damage ligaments and the joint capsule. Articular changes occur from the abnormal composition of synovial fluid, which damages the hyaline cartilage. Collapse of a femoral or tibial condyle can result from cyst formation in the bony structures. As the cartilage wears down, crepitus is evident throughout range of motion.

Early in the rheumatoid process, near symmetrical involvement is seen in the mediolateral and patellofemoral components. A knee flexion contracture is frequently seen as slight flexion decreases joint stress. This flexion is maintained by a muscle spasm of the hamstrings. In knee flexion, the proximal tibia is posterior to the distal femur. With severe contractures, the resultant subluxation can approximate a posterior tibial dislocation. This only occurs to this profound extent in a non-ambulatory patient. If a patient is still walking, seldom is there limitation of motion greater than 20° to 30°. With a slight flexion contracture, there is usually no component of angulation in the frontal plane. Therefore, the medial collateral and lateral collateral ligaments are not altered. However, the posterior joint is shortened and the quadriceps are weakened from prolonged elongation.[18]

As the rheumatoid changes progress, joint erosion no longer occurs symmetrically and mediolateral instability is seen. Usually this results in a valgus deformity. The muscle spasm then includes the tensor fascia lata which further pulls the tibia laterally on the femur. Additionally, tibial external rotation occurs in more than 50 percent of the patients with moderate to severe rheumatoid knee changes. This causes a shortening of all lateral joint structures and a permanent lengthening and weakening of medial structures, particularly with weight bearing.

More severe articular change is seen with prolonged maintenance of these abnormal joint positions. Anterior glide at the tibia is blocked by an actual bony ridge formed transversely on the distal femur. Disuse osteoporosis can develop as pain limits activity with resultant fractures. The loss of hyaline cartilage can be quite severe with crepitation experienced in any weight bearing position.[19]

The interaction of the foot and knee must be assessed. A pronated foot medially deviates the ground reaction force in standing and places a valgus stress on the knee. Conversely, genu valgus can cause foot pronation as a plantigrade foot position is attempted (Fig. 7-2).[20]

During gait, restriction of motion at the knee decreases the velocity and increases the energy expenditure. More work is required in the acceleration period of swing phase to bring the lower extremity forward. Kettlecamp looked at the gait patterns of 41 patients with rheumatoid arthritis and knee involvement.[21] This study confirmed that range of motion, cadence, and stride length are all decreased in these patients. They used 25 percent of the available knee range of motion, compared to 46 percent used normally. Cadence dropped to 72.5 steps per minute from the 109 to 120 steps per minute normally seen. Stride length was shorted by approximately 50 percent. Stauffer et al carried out another biomechanical gait analysis study, including patients with rheumatoid arthritis and knee involvement.[22] This showed the walking velocity to be 36 percent of normal and there was a 45 percent reduction of hamstring contraction and 23 percent reduction of quadriceps contraction during gait.

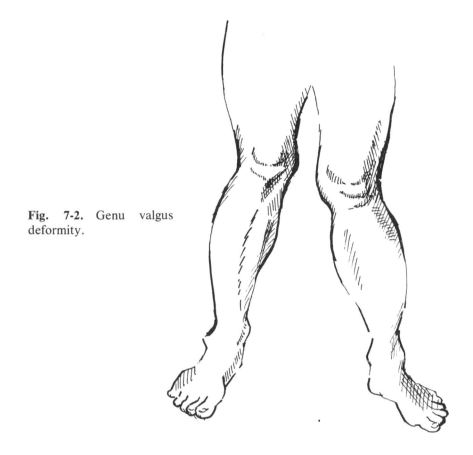

Fig. 7-2. Genu valgus deformity.

The Hip

The frequency of hip involvement in rheumatoid arthritis varies with the length of time a person has had the disease. Early in the clinical course hips are involved in only 5 to 10 percent of the patients, while with more advanced rheumatoid arthritis 50 percent of the patients showed changes in the hip.[16]

Changes at the femoral acetabular joint are clearly evidenced by alterations in gait and the ability to accomplish activities of daily living. This limitation is particularly seen in those tasks dealing with personal hygiene. Range of motion becomes limited, primarily in extension and abduction. This restriction can be from muscle spasm and/or joint structural changes.

The pelvis must be stabilized for accurate measurement of hip range of motion. Joint tenderness can often be palpated at the posterior/superior aspect of the trochanter where the gluteal muscles attach, the adductor attachment to the ischium, and/or the iliopectineal region.[23] This generally occurs with tendinitis or a tension myalgia syndrome. Inflammation can occur within the hip joint, although the large muscle mass in this area makes it difficult to clearly assess. If swelling is visible, it is seen in the groin or femoral triangle. If trochanteric bursitis is present, tenderness can be palpated directly over the greater trochanteric head. In severe and rare cases, the bony consequences can be substantial. Osteoporosis can become so advanced that the femoral head penetrates the acetabulum. Avascular necrosis of the femoral head can cause collapse of this area and a true leg length discrepancy.

During the stance phase, the gait pattern of a patient with hip pain will reveal decreased time in single limb stance, lateral trunk flexion towards the affected side, and a contralateral dropped pelvis with weight bearing. If an assistive device is used, considerable relief can be obtained. The forces on the hip from the abductor muscles and gravity can be reduced by 30 percent if a standard cane is used on the contralateral side.[24] To accomplish this the load applied to the cane can be relatively small. This has been measured in three studies and found to be between 4 and 15 kg.[24,25] However, while a cane beneficially lowers the compressive force on the hip, it alters the direction of that force. The new vertical force is concentrated on the superior surface of the femoral head and outer rim of the acetabulum which is less suitable for weight bearing.[1]

TYPICAL GAIT PATTERNS WITH RHEUMATOID ARTHRITIS

The common deformities of the lower extremity joints in a patient with rheumatoid arthritis biomechanically alter the kinetics and kinematics involved in gait. An acute exacerbation of any lower extremity joint will cause decreased stance time on that leg. The forefoot and midfoot deformities primarily alter the stance phase. With forefoot change, there is diminished roll-off at terminal stance, apropulsive progression at the end of stance and decreased balance in single limb support. Additionally, hallux valgus causes a lateral and posterior weight shift in late stance and a late heel rise. Deformity in the subtalar joint will typically be evident by a pronated foot in weight bearing, shuffled progression with lack of a clear heel-toe pattern, decreased step length, initial contact with the medial border of the foot, and increased double support time.[13] Also seen are late heel rise, plantarflexion of the ipsilateral lower extremity during swing phase,[26] and possible genu valgus with weight bearing.[20] A patient with a painful heel from plantar fasciitis or a heel spur will use a toe-heel pattern, have no heel contact in stance phase, decreased stride length and velocity, swing phase ankle plantarflexion and increased hip flexion, and a decreased step length of the contralateral limb. Knee involvement has been looked at in several gait studies.[21,22] Normally, a decrease in knee range of motion, cadence, and stride length is seen. Since about 50 percent of the knee flexion is used compared to normal, there is a change in swing phase in addition to stance phase. Because the amount of knee flexion may not be sufficient to clear the foot in limb advancement, a steppage or circumducted gait pattern may be seen. If a patient with hip pain and radiographic changes at the hip is ambulating without assistive devices, an antalgic pattern is usually seen. A compensated or uncompensated Trendelenburg gait pattern is also likely to reduce compressive loads on the hip.[1]

COMMON PATHOPHYSIOLOGIC CHANGES IN OTHER FORMS OF ARTHRITIS IN THE LOWER EXTREMITIES AND RESULTANT FUNCTIONAL CHANGES

Osteoarthritis, or degenerative joint disease, is more commonly seen in the general population than rheumatoid arthritis. As our life expectancy increases, so too will the incidence of osteoarthritis. Although it can be as functionally limiting as rheumatoid arthritis, this rarely occurs. Major differences between the two pathologies are that osteoarthritis is unilateral, noninflammatory, and not a systemic disease. Osteoarthritis affects the weight bearing joints; therefore, the lower extremity joints and spine are the sites of usual involvement. When assistive gait devices are used, the upper extremity joints also share weight bearing and are likely to show degenerative changes. Pathologically, there is a progressive deterioration and loss of articular cartilage. The margins of the joints and the subchondral bone change, with an eventual sclerosis of the subchondral bone. Clinically, patients experience a slowly developing joint pain, stiffness, enlargement of joint size, and limitation of motion. A secondary synovitis is often seen, resulting in a hot, swollen joint as is seen in rheumatoid arthritis. Joint hypermobility can occur because of the narrowed joint space and resultant ligamentous laxity. As the disease progresses there is often prolific marginal osteophyte formation and cyst formation. This causes a marked protective decrease in range of motion (ROM) and joint stiffness will occur. Actual ankylosis is not common except in patients with a particular type of osteoarthritis known as erosive inflammatory osteoarthritis. This primarily occurs in the hands.

Degenerative joint disease of the spine results from involvement of the weight bearing areas here which include the intervertebral discs and the facet joints. This leads to what is commonly known as mechanical low back pain. There can be a radicular component due to compression of a nerve root from spur formation.

Osteoarthritic changes at the hip cause pain in the groin, buttocks, or along a sciatic distribution due to close proximity of the sciatic nerve to the hip joint. Radiographs show most deterioration along the superior pole of the femoral head because this is the area of most weight bearing. A Trendelenburg gait pattern will be seen, either compensated or uncompensated, depending on the status of the other hip. A hip flexion contracture may be present, which causes an apparent leg length discrepancy when the patient is upright. Limitation of motion primarily occurs in internal rotation and extension. Involvement at the hip is the most disabling form of osteoarthritis although it is not as common as osteoarthritis of the knee. Degenerative joint disease is commonly seen at the knee. The medial joint compartment, which bears most of the weight in ambulation, is the site of most deterioration. This results in a genu varus de-

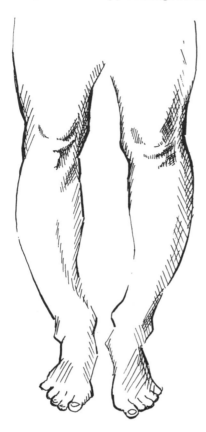

Fig. 7-3. Genu varus deformity.

formity (Fig. 7-3). Chondromalacia patella is a condition frequently seen in young adults. This is a softening and erosion of the patellar articular cartilage; more severe osteoarthritic changes can follow. Patients with this problem will complain of pain whenever the patella is compressed, as occurs with weight bearing on a flexed knee. At the ankle the tibiotalar joint, which is the primary site of weight bearing, is most involved. This results in decreased plantar and dorsiflexion of the ankle. In the forefoot the metatarsophalangeal joint of the great toe shows most degeneration. It is this toe which bears 50 percent of the weight bearing of the five toes during ambulation. Rigidity of this toe will shorten the stride length of the opposite lower extremity in gait, as the patient will hesitate to bear weight on the forefoot requiring flexion of this toe.

Much less commonly seen are the diseases of gout, pseudogout or chondrocalcinosis, and Reiter's syndrome. These are included here as each can have significant lower extremity involvement to greatly alter mobility. Gout typically affects the first metatarsophalangeal joint and the tarsal joints of the foot, the ankle, and the knee. Involvement of the great toe occurs in 75 percent or more of all patients. Fortunately, this form of arthritis is now well controlled with medication and diet, and periods of exacerbation should be short-lived. During an acute phase rest is mandatory. Generally the severe pain associated with this will dictate a non-weight bearing or bed rest status. Pseudogout characteristically affects the knees, spine, hips, and ankles, in addition to some upper extremity joints. If not previously diagnosed, an exacerbation of pseudogout at the knee can mimic a gout attack or medial meniscus tear. The acute attacks are marked by inflammation and can last several days or longer. They are generally less painful than true gouty arthritis. The attacks are often provocated by surgery or trauma. Reiter's syndrome can cause pain at the base of the heel. This may result from a subcalcaneal bursitis or plantar fasciitis or, in later stages, calcaneal periostitis with spur formation. To reduce stress on the calcaneus, shock absorption should be maximally provided by the shoe, thus a cushioned heel is mandatory. The velocity of gait may need to be decreased to diminish the ground reaction force at heel strike.

COMPONENTS OF REHABILITATION

Rest

During periods of acute exacerbation of arthritis, the major goals of treatment are to reduce inflammation and relieve pain. This is accomplished with rest, reduction of harmful mechanical stresses, and appropriate medication.[27] When swelling is noted in lower extremity joints, all weight bearing on those joints should be discouraged until acute inflammation subsides. Proper positioning during this rest is of utmost importance to maintain range of motion. If resting splints are being used, they should be removed daily for active assistive range of motion exercises. It is important to avoid the positions of typical joint contractures. Therefore, at the hip the rest position should not be one of flexion and external rotation; the knee should not be held in flexion, and the foot should be supported in a neutral position. Thermal and/or electrical modalities may be used prior to exercises to relieve pain and inhibitory muscle spasm, allowing fullest excursion in exercise. Both heat and cold reduce muscle spindle activities.[28] Isometric muscle contractions of the quadriceps and gluteal muscles should be done if a patient is on bedrest, to minimize the effects of diffuse muscle atrophy.[29]

Assistive Gait Devices

As the patient enters the subacute phase of rehabilitation, partial weight bearing ambulation can be started. Assistive gait devices must be wisely chosen with consideration given to the status of the upper extremity joints. As these devices decrease stress on joints of the legs, they convert the joints of the upper extremities to a weight bearing status. The amount of deformity and function in the arms will dictate the type of device chosen. Continuous monitoring of the upper extremities will be necessary during use of the device. Specific therapeutic intervention may be required to strengthen the shoulder and elbow extensors in preparation for gait. If possible, the weight bearing should be distributed over as broad an area as possible, as is done with platform walkers or crutches, and broad handled canes.

Energy Considerations

The energy required for ambulation increases as the upper extremities are required to work, the speed is increased, and the determinants of gait are lost or compromised. Therefore, any time the upper extremities are used for weight bearing, and/or a lower extremity joint is restricted in motion, the work load for the person is increased. If a patient is deconditioned or has evidence of cardiopulmonary disease, consideration should be given to gradual aerobic conditioning as a component of, or in addition to, gait training.

Shoes

Appropriate shoe wear can have a significant influence on the ambulatory status of a patient with arthritis involving the joints of the feet and ankles. As already discussed, joint instability is the primary problem altering function. The shoe, and orthotic devices when needed, should augment joint stability. Furthermore, they should decrease weight bearing loads on vulnerable areas of deformity and transfer these forces to more suitable areas. Desirable qualities in a shoe include adequate width and depth, a soft upper, a cushion sole, a low heel, a longitudinal arch support, and a firm medial counter.[19] As many rheumatoid deformities do not become evident until weight bearing, the shoe must be fit in the weight bearing position. For most patients these qualifications are met in commercially available shoes of the standard oxford type. Two specific orthopedic lasts are also available and can accommodate some deformities. Constriction of hallux valgus can be avoided with a bunion last providing a wide fore part, or a combination last with a wide fore part and relatively narrow heel. Extra depth shoes can also be purchased allowing room for toe deformities and/or an orthotic foot device. Some patients will require custom-made shoes. These are not meant to correct existing deformities, but do prolong ambulation by providing external stability and the most suitable weight bearing patterns for an individual.

Orthotics

Orthotics can be effectively used for the foot, ankle, and knee, and to a lesser degree at the hip. One classification system for orthotic devices divides them into either functional or balance types. The former stabilizes a body part during function of that area, and/or a distal segment, while the latter orthosis distributes pressure. A functional orthosis must therefore be sufficiently rigid to restrict unwanted motion, and is used during all weight bearing activities. This would be appropriate at the foot, ankle and knee. Examples of balance orthoses are modifications of the soles of the shoe, which redistribute stress and the ground reaction force by changing the position of the foot in relation to the ground. Metatarsal bars are used to decrease weight bearing on painful and/or subluxed metatarsal heads. Correct placement of these bars proximal to the metatarsal heads is crucial to their effectiveness. When forefoot weight bearing is difficult, a rigid rocker bar can be used to decrease metatarsal phalangeal flexion and provide a smooth roll to toe off. Plantigrade stability can be enhanced by use of medial or lateral heel flanges. Other types of balance orthoses can be placed within the shoe and are generally made of compliant materials which greatly enhance comfort by reducing the ground reaction force.[8] Although not frequently seen, a knee-ankle-foot orthosis with either an ischial weight bearing ring or a quadrilateral plastic thigh socket can be used to alleviate hip pain in ambulation. To effectively transmit body weight and bypass the hip, all distal joint range of motion must be restricted. This drastically increases the energy expenditure required for ambulation.[1] Therefore, although the orthosis relieves hip pain, ambulation becomes quite difficult with it on and is seldom used.

The field of orthotics has made many advances as the ability for biomechanical analysis of joints improves, and stronger and lighter materials are produced. Traditionally, patient compliance with any orthotic larger than a foot orthosis is poor. Most patients with rheumatoid arthritis have significant difficulty in fine hand tasks and donning a large orthotic device can be a difficult, if not impossible chore. Fortunately, correcting malalignment at a distal joint may be all that is needed to properly align and increase stability at a more proximal joint.

Exercise

Specific exercise programs should be a part of the overall rehabilitation regimen of any patient diagnosed as having arthritis. A primary function of the lower extremity joints is that of bearing body weight, and exercises here should be done to increase and/or maintain strength, primarily in extensor muscle groups. This is most easily done isometrically as the joint is held stable while muscular forces are increased. If muscle strength is maintained, normal weight bearing paths are also maintained. At the hip, both the gluteus maximus and medius should be strengthened while the hip flexor length must be maintained. The knee usually requires strengthening of the quadriceps and stretching of the hamstrings. Little can be strengthened at the ankle and foot to enhance stability, but full range of motion should be maintained to allow normal transfers of force in all planes. As previously mentioned, the upper extremity strength must be sufficient to allow proper use of assistive gait devices when needed.

Devices Needed to Increase Mobility

Fortunately, few patients with arthritis will become so functionally limited that a state of wheelchair dependency is reached. When required, the chair must be prescribed for the individual with consideration given to his/her size, lifestyle, and upper extremity abilities. Components that may be helpful include a lightweight model, elevating and removable foot rests to decrease the chance of knee flexion contractures, a seat cushion to decrease ischial pressure and raise the seat height to help in standing, a brake extension lever, and oblique projections on the wheel rims to accommodate diminished hand function.[19] Other devices frequently considered for use with the patient with rheumatoid arthritis include an elevated toilet seat, tub railings, a tub seat, chair cushions to elevate the seat height, long handled mirrors, long handled reachers, and modifications in the house to allow activities of daily living to be done at mid-ranges rather than the extremes.

Postoperative Considerations

Orthopedic surgical advances have occurred in all types of reconstructive surgery. Specific rehabilitation programs vary greatly at each joint and with each procedure. It is important that the therapist be aware of mechanical alterations occurring during surgery, so that the functional status can be maximally achieved. All of the previously mentioned considerations of assistive gait devices, modalities, exercise, and resting positions have an important role in this phase of rehabilitation.

REFERENCES

1. Inman VT, Ralston HJ, Todd F: Human Walking. Williams & Wilkins, Baltimore, 1981
2. Wright, DG, Desai SM, Henderson WH: Action of subtalar and ankle joint complex during the stance phase of walking. J Bone Joint Surg 46A 2:361, 1964
3. Nordin M, Frankel VH: Biomechanics of the knee. p. 113. In Frankel VH, Nordin M (eds): Basic Biomechanics of the Skeletal System, Lea & Febiger, Philadelphia, 1980
4. Laubenthal KN, Smidt GL, Kettelkamp DB: A quantitative analysis of knee motion during activities of daily living. Phys Ther 52:34, 1972
5. Nordin M, Frankel VH: Biomechanics of the hip. p. 149. In Frankel VH, Nordin M (eds): Basic Biomechanics of the Skeletal System. Lea & Febiger, Philadelphia, 1980
6. Paul JP: forces at the hip joint. PhD thesis, University of Chicago, Chicago, 1967
7. Poss R, Sledge CB: Surgery of the hip in rheumatoid arthritis. p. 1960. In Kelly WN, Harris ED, Ruddy S, Sledge CB (eds): Textbook of Rheumatology. WB Saunders, Philadelphia, 1981

8. Wood B: The painful foot. p. 472. In Kelley WN, Harris ED, Ruddy S, Sledge CB (eds): Textbook of Rheumatology. WB Saunders, Philadelphia, 1981

9. Mann RA, Coughlin MJ: The rheumatoid foot: Review of literature and method of treatment. Orthop Rev 8:105, 1979

10. Calabro JJ: A critical evaluation of the diagnostic features of the feet in rheumatoid arthritis. Arthritis Rheum 5:19, 1962

11. Thomas WH: Reconstructive surgery and rehabilitation of the ankle and foot. p. 1999. In Kelley WN, Harris ED, Ruddy S, Sledge CB (eds): Textbook of Rheumatology. WB Saunders, Philadelphia, 1981

12. Jacoby RK, Jayson MIV, Cosh JA: Onset early stages and prognosis of rheumatoid arthritis: A clinical study of 100 patients with 11 year follow up. Br Med J 2:96, 1973

13. DiMonte P, Light H: Pathomechanics, gait deviations and treatment of the rheumatoid foot. Phys Ther 62:1148, 1982

14. King J, Burke D, Freeman MAR: The incidence of pain in the rheumatoid hindfoot and the significance of calcaneofibular impingement. Int Orthop 2:255, 1978

15. Vidigal E, Jacoby RK, Dixon ASt. J et al: The foot in chronic rheumatoid arthritis. Ann Rheum Dis 34:392, 1975

16. McKenna F, Wright V: Clinical Manifestations. p. 283. In Utsinger PD, Zvaifler NJ, Ehrlich GE (eds): Rheumatoid Arthritis. JB Lippincott, Philadelphia, 1985

17. Potter TA: Mechanisms of deformity of the rheumatoid arthritic knee. Surg Clin North Am 49:889, 1969

18. Insall J: Reconstructive surgery and rehabilitation of the knee. p. 1980. In Kelley WN, Harris ED, Ruddy S, Sledge CB (eds): Textbook of Rheumatology, WB Saunders, Philadelphia, 1981

19. Slack D, Levine P, Banwell B, Utsinger PD: Physical medicine and rehabilitation. p. 711. In Utsinger PD, Zvaifler NJ, Ehrlich GE (eds): Rheumatoid Arthritis. JB Lippincott, Philadelphia, 1985

20. Shields MN, Ward JR: Treatment of related knee-ankle-foot deformities in rheumatoid arthritis. Phys Ther 46:600, 1966

21. Kettlekamp DB, Leaverton PE, Misol S: Gait characteristics of the rheumatoid knee. Arch Surg 104:30, 1972

22. Stauffer RN, Chad EYS, Gyory AN: Biomechanical gait analysis of the diseased knee joint. CORR 126:246, 1977

23. Vollertsen RS, Hunder GG: Approach to the patient and examination of the musculoskeletal system. p. 000. In Utsinger PD, Zvaifler NJ, Ehrlich GE (eds): Rheumatoid Arthritis. JB Lippincott, Philadelphia, 1985

24. Bergmann G, Kolbel R, Rauschenboch N, Rohlmann A: Crutch walking and hip mechanics. Proc British Orthopaedic Research Society meeting, Now 1977. J Bone Joint Surgery 60B:281, 1978

25. Murray MP, Seireg AH, Scholz RC. A survey of the time, magnitude and orientation of forces applied to walking sticks by disabled men. Am J Phys Med 48:1, 1969

26. Marshall RN, Meyers DB, Palmer DG: Disturbance of gait due to rheumatoid disease. J Rheumatol 7:617, 1980

27. Navarro AH: Physical therapy in the management of rheumatoid arthritis. Clin Rheumatol Pract 1:125, 1983

28. Lehmann JF, Warren CG, Scham SM: Therapeutic heat and cold. Clin Orthop 99:207, 1974

29. Machover S, Sapecky AJ: Effect of isometric exercise on the quadriceps muscle in patients with rheumatoid arthritis. Arch Phys Med Rehabil 47:737, 1966

8 | Splinting and Joint Protection

Peggy T. McKnight

Satisfactory management of the patient with rheumatoid disease depends on many factors, including the therapeutic effects of drugs and the use of a conservative treatment regimen to maintain or increase the patient's functional capacity. Components of this regimen may include exercise and therapeutic activities, the use of adaptive and assistive devices, the local application of heat or cold, the use of whirlpool, ultrasound, and electrical modalities, and a program that incorporates splinting and protection of the inflamed joints.

Although the effects of splinting and joint protection techniques are well known and have been widely documented, controversy continues to exist over the relative values of either treatment modality. The intent of this chapter is to review general principles of splinting and joint protection and to discuss the value of these modalities in the care of the rheumatic disease patient.

This chapter is divided into two sections. The first section will discuss the indications and methods for splinting a variety of common rheumatologic disorders. For the purpose of this section, splints will be classified into three types:

Splints to relieve pain and inflammation
Splints to prevent or correct deformity
Splints to improve function

The principles of joint protection and energy conservation will be discussed in the second section. Throughout both sections, an attempt has been made to condense what is important based on a review of the literature and the author's experience. It is hoped that this chapter will not only provide answers to some questions, but also raise questions for future investigation. To begin, we will briefly review the disease process as it exists in the patient with rheumatoid arthritis, so as to provide a model for understanding the importance of splinting and joint protection in a comprehensive treatment program.

Rheumatoid arthritis is thought to be an autoimmune disease in which the patient manufactures antibodies, with the resulting inflammatory reaction occurring principally in the synovial tissue of joints and tendons as well as ligaments. This inflammation leads to stretching of the supporting joint capsule and ligaments surrounding the joint, resulting in weakness and joint damage.[1] In later stages of the disease process, the synovium invades and erodes the articular cartilage and the subchondral bone, eventually causing joint destruction and deformity.

Deformity of the hands occurs in at least one quarter of the cases of rheumatoid arthritis.[2] Although these deformities vary, wrist flexion deformity, secondary to subluxation of the carpal bones and resulting in an imbalance of the long flexor and extensor tendons to the digits, is frequently seen. Other common deformities include flexion contracture of the metacarpophalangeal (MCP) joints with volar subluxation and ulnar deviation, and swan neck or boutonnière deformities of the fingers.

The course of rheumatoid arthritis is variable and may be divided into three phases. In the acute phase, the symptoms of joint inflammation (pain, tenderness, swelling, and limitation of joint motion) are the most severe. In the subacute phase, the acute symptoms of joint inflammation are present though less intense, and deformities resulting from instability of the joints occur. The final or chronic stage is characterized by joint destruction and, occasionally, ankylosis. The use of splinting and joint protection principles are of value when used appropriately throughout the various stages of the disease process and may be useful in managing a variety of common rheumatologic problems.

SPLINTING

Splinting for Relief of Pain and Inflammation

In the opinion of most physicians and therapists, the use of splints is of value in the management of patients with the acute, inflammatory stage of rheumatoid arthritis. Several studies have documented the beneficial effects of splinting for pain relief, decrease of muscle spasm, and decrease of disease activity.[3–12] A study by Zoeckler in 1969 found that 63 percent of the patients who regularly wore splints noted relief of pain and stiffness, while patients who did not regularly wear splints did not.[13] In another study by Biddulph, the efficacy of the Futuro wrist splint for eight patients with rheumatoid arthritis found 75 percent noted relief of night pain and 87.5 percent noted functional improvement.[12] In addition, Swanson,[2] Flatt,[3] and Rotstein[5] advocate the use of splints for pain relief and decrease of inflammation.

Controversy exists regarding the degree of immobilization needed to reduce active disease process and whether immobilization may contribute to decreased range of motion, reduced muscle strength, atrophy, and eventual ankylosis. A study by Gault and Spyker suggests that immobilization for a 3– week period is beneficial and does not result in permanent decrease of motion range or loss of muscle strength in patients with acute rheumatoid arthritis (ARA) Stage I, II, and early Stage III rheumatoid arthritis joints.[10]

In another study, published in 1963, Partridge and Duthie compared two groups of patients.[9] One group was confined to bed for 4 weeks and plaster splints were applied to the arms and legs, immobilizing the four major joints except the shoulders and hips. Patients in the control group were confined to bed for 4 weeks but were allowed up for toilet purposes. This group received splints for all four joints, but the splints were removed two times daily for exercise. Following the 4-week period, complete immobilization was terminated in the first group, and both groups received the exercise treatments. Results indicated improvement in range of motion and functional capacity in both groups, and no joint ankylosis occurred in any patient during the course of the study. Diminution of disease activity was greatest in the group of patients who were completely immobilized, suggesting complete immobilization for limited time periods can be used safely and efficaciously in the management of rheumatoid arthritis. In yet another study, Harris found no significant differences in motion range of the knee joint with utilization of intermittent versus continuous immobilization.[14]

Overall, the consensus is that immobilization from 2 to 4 weeks can be safely used to control pain, muscle spasm, and disease activity during the acute stage of rheumatoid arthritis without risk of the development of joint contractures or ankylosis.[9–11,15]

Volar Resting Splints

Goals

Relieve pain
Reduce inflammation
Maintain proper alignment of joints
Support and protect soft tissues and structures
Counterbalance the pull of flexor muscles
Improve function

Treatment Principles.   The wrist should be splinted in 20° to 30° of extension and in 10° of ulnar deviation. The MCP joints should be flexed to approximately 45° to preserve the length of the collateral ligaments.[16–18] The thumb should be positioned in abduction and opposition (Figs. 8-1 and 8-2).

Traditionally, resting splints have been applied at night and removed during the day to permit hand function. If resting splints are used at night for both hands, they should be alternately worn to permit hand function necessary for

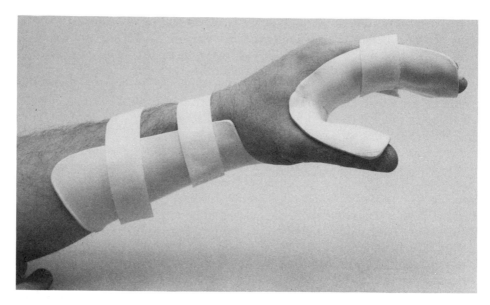

Fig. 8-1. Volar resting splint provides passive immobilization of the wrist and fingers.

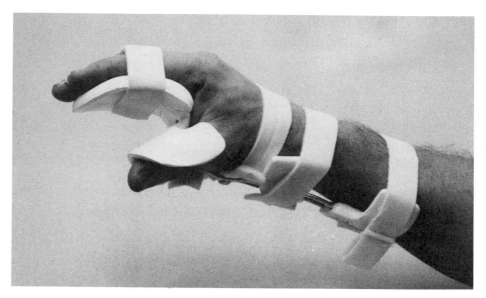

Fig. 8-2. Volar wire foam wrist and finger orthosis provide passive immobilization of the wrist and fingers.

toileting purposes. Non-compliance with the wearing of these splints has been attributed by patients to their clumsiness and patient inability to perform such nighttime tasks as toileting. In a recent study by Feinburg, compliance with wearing full hand resting splints was shown to be 62 percent.[19]

Resting splints are commercially available or may be fabricated out of high or low temperature splinting materials.

The Static Wrist and MCP Stabilization Splint

Goals

Relieve pain
Relieve inflammation
Maintain proper alignment of joints
Counterbalance the pull of flexor muscles
Support and protect soft tissues and structures
Improve function
Counteract intrinsic tightness

Treatment Principles.   The wrist should be splinted in 20° to 30° of extension and 10° of ulnar deviation. The MCP joints should be splinted in 0° of extension and the splint should extend past the MCP joints but allow PIP joint flexion (Fig. 8-3).

This type of splint is recommended for patients who present with coexisting synovitis of the wrist and MCP joints; the use of a splint which immobilizes only the wrist may create additional stress to the MCP joints.[16,18] This splint is also recommended for wear during exercise or activity for patients with intrinsic muscle tightness.[16] If worn during the day, patients should be cautioned that it will limit hand function requiring grasp.

This splint may be fabricated with high or low temperature splinting materials.

Static Wrist Splints

Goals

Relieve pain
Relieve inflammation
Relieve symptoms of carpal tunnel syndrome
Provide stability of a subluxed wrist
Improve grip strength
Improve function

Treatment Principles.   The wrist should be splinted in 20° to 30° of extension and the splint should extend up to the distal palmar crease to allow full thumb opposition and finger motion.

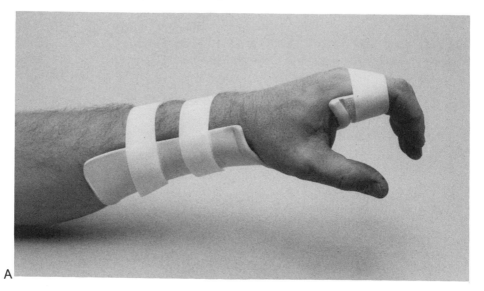

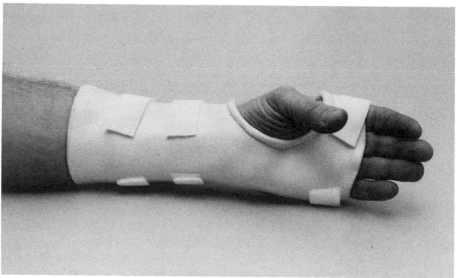

Fig. 8-3. (A,B) Static wrist and metacarpophalangeal stabilization splint provide immobilization of the wrist and metacarpophalangeal joints.

The wrist is considered the keystone of the hand. Therefore, wrist stability without pain is necessary for normal hand function, as instability and weakness lead to weak grasp. Traditionally, static wrist splints have been recommended for wear during the day, when a patient is performing activities which cause wrist stress or pain. These splints may also be worn at night for pain relief.[6,20]

Static splints may be fabricated with thermoplastic materials or are com-

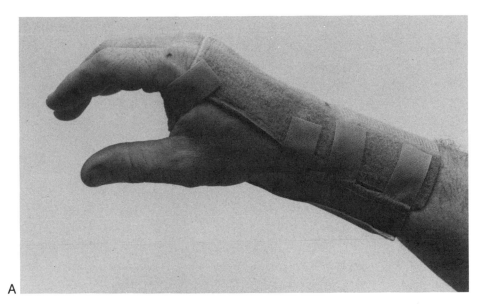

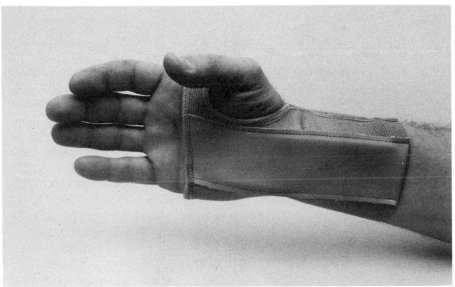

Fig. 8-4. (A,B) Futuro wrist splint supports the wrist in the desired position and allows full finger motion and thumb opposition.

mercially available. Two commercially available wrist splints are the Futuro (Fig. 8-4) and the Currie (Fig. 8-5). Commercially available splints have the advantage of being economical and efficient, particularly for patients suffering from carpal tunnel syndrome.[15,21] They also seem to be easier to wear when performing certain types of grasp activities, such as holding onto crutches or

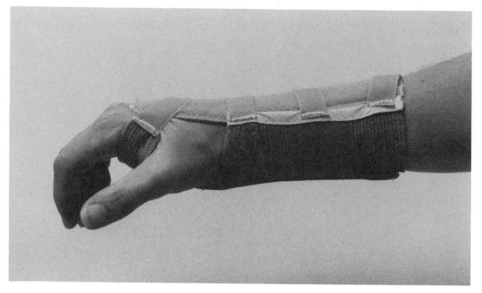

Fig. 8-5. Currie wrist splint supports the wrist in the desired position and allows full finger motion and thumb opposition.

canes. Cosmetic acceptability also seems greater with the commercially available splints. In many cases, however, commercially available splints require multiple adjustments to ensure proper fit and may cause pressure and irritation over the ulnar styloid.

When deciding between a thermoplastic and a commercially available splint, other factors should be considered. According to Melvin, the utilization of a static splint for immobilization of the wrist can create additional stress to the MCP joints[1] (Fig. 8-6). However, the more flexible the wrist splint, the less force will be transferred. The Futuro wrist splint, which is flexible and allows up to 50° of wrist flexion and extension, may, therefore, be advisable for patients with MCP synovitis.[1,16] However, for patients with moderate to severe wrist synovitis or wrist subluxation, the stronger, thermoplastic wrist splint is the more effective treatment. In all cases, utilization of static wrist splints requires that the therapist monitor MCP synovitis so as to not aggravate this condition.[16]

Static Wrist Splint with Thumb Attachment

Goals

Relieve pain
Relieve inflammation

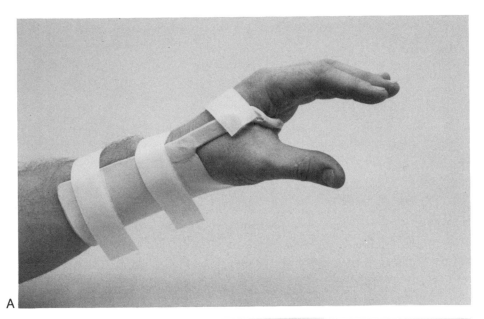

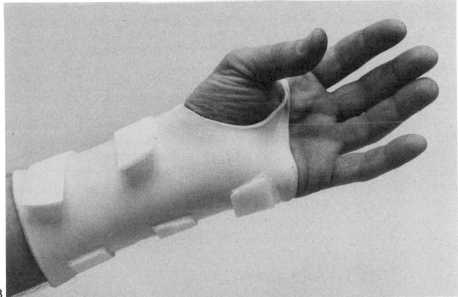

Fig. 8-6. (A,B)   Static wrist splint supports the wrist in the desired position and allows full finger motion and thumb opposition.

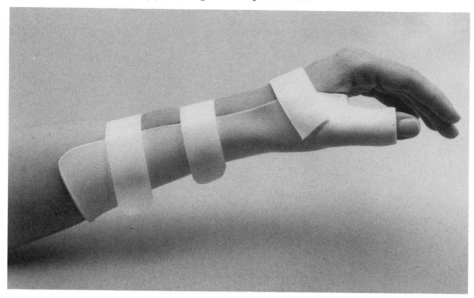

Fig. 8-7.   Static wrist splint with thumb attachment immobilizes the wrist, carpome-tacarpal, and metacarpophalangeal joints, leaving the interphalangeal joint free to pinch.

> Relieve symptoms of DeQuervain's disease
> Provide stability
> Improve function

Treatment Principles.   The wrist should be splinted in 20° to 30° of extension and the thumb splinted in abduction to allow finger tip prehension (Fig. 8-7).

Thumb involvement is frequently encountered in the rheumatic disease patient. In patients with osteoarthritis, the carpometacarpal (CMC) joint of the thumb may be affected and in patients with rheumatoid arthritis, synovitis may involve the CMC and MCP joints.[1,15] In both groups of patients, thumb involvement may result in pain, instability, and reduced hand function. This splint effectively provides stability and pain relief for the thumb when worn during activities requiring pinch and also provides stability to the wrist.[22] However, some patients report compromise of mobility and hand function with this type of splint.

Short Static Thumb Splint

Goals

Relieve pain
Relieve inflammation

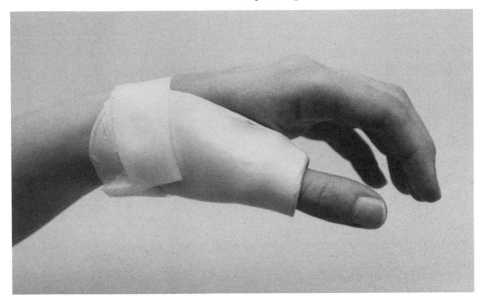

Fig. 8-8. Short static thumb splint immobilizes the metacarpophalangeal joint and provides partial immobilization of the carpometacarpophalangeal joint. It allows interphalangeal joint mobility. The thumb should be splinted in abduction.

Provide stability
Improve function

Treatment Principles.   The short static thumb splint is not generally recommended for patients with multiple joint involvement. Although it does not completely restrict thumb CMC joint mobility, it can serve to diminish pain.[1] This splint is commercially available or may be fabricated out of high or low temperature splinting material (Fig. 8-8). For patients with severe CMC joint involvement, the wrist splint with thumb attachment is recommended.

Stretch Gloves

Goals

Relieve pain
Relieve stiffness
Decrease swelling

Treatment Principles.   Night time use of stretch gloves has been shown to be effective for the symptomatic treatment of arthritis.[23-26] Askari et al[23] and Ehrlich et al[24] found that the external compression from stretch gloves was effective in reducing night pain and morning stiffness in the hands of patients

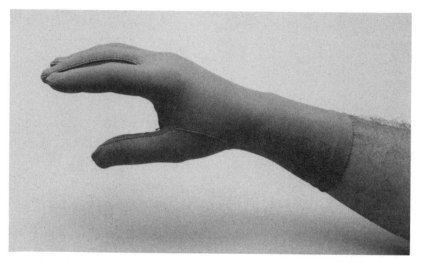

Fig. 8-9.   Stretch gloves provide external compression for relief of pain, stiffness, and swelling.

with arthritis. Similarly, Culic et al[25] and Swezey et al[26] reported that these gloves reduced ring size in patients with rheumatoid arthritis. Stretch gloves are commercially available, inexpensive, and easy to apply (Fig. 8-9).

Air Compression Splints

Goals

Relieve pain
Relieve stiffness
Decrease swelling
Improve grip strength
Improve range of motion

Treatment Principles.   There has been one published report of an uncontrolled study on the use of the static air compression splint for symptomatic relief of hand symptoms in patients with rheumatoid arthritis.[27] The air splint, which permits the simultaneous application of a constant, uniform external pressure, was effective in reducing pain, stiffness, and swelling, and improving strength and motion in the hands of 30 patients with rheumatoid arthritis.

These results indicate that air splint treatments can promote both objective and subjective improvement in the symptoms of rheumatoid synovitis of the hands, and it appears to be a significant addition to the management of patients with rheumatoid arthritis (Fig. 8-10). The air splint, which is commercially available, is inexpensive and easy to use.

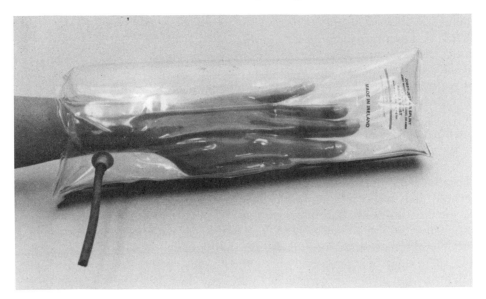

Fig. 8-10. Air compression splint provides external compression for relief of inflammation.

Treatment Principles for the Use of Cervical Orthoses

Cervical spine involvement is frequently found in patients with rheumatoid arthritis, resulting in symptoms of pain, muscle spasm, paresthesia, and weakness. Progressive involvement commonly leads to subluxation of the first and second cervical vertebrae, and may result in spinal cord compression. Subluxation of the low cervical spine may also occur, producing symptoms of nerve root compression, resulting in radiation of pain to the upper extremity.

While the main objectives of splinting are to alleviate pain, control muscle spasm, and to restrict neck mobility, the effectiveness of cervical orthoses for restricting neck mobility has not been well proven. Colachis and associates studied the effectiveness of the soft sponge collar, chin-piece collar, and Queen-Anne collar.[28] They concluded that the soft collar did not restrict flexion of the cervical spine and only slightly restricted extension. The chin-piece and Queen-Anne collars limited flexion and extension; however, no statistical analysis of the data was done. In another study by Hartman and associates, the effectiveness of a soft collar, Thomas collar, four-poster, long two-poster and Guilford two-brace was evaluated.[29] They concluded that the soft collar provided immobilization of 5 to 10 percent, the Thomas collar about 75 percent decrease of flexion-extension, the four-poster 80 to 85 percent, the long two-poster 90 to 95 percent and the Guilford two-poster 95 percent.

Fisher and associates studied the effectiveness of the polyethylene Camp plastic collar, the plastazote Philadelphia collar, the four-poster orthosis, and the sternal occipital mandibular immobilization (SOMI) orthosis to determine their effectiveness in limiting flexion and extension of the cervical spine.[30] The SOMI orthosis provided the best immobilization for preventing flexion of the entire cervical spine. The four-poster orthosis provided the best immobilization of all vertebral levels in preventing extension except at 0-C1 and C1-C2. The polyethylene Camp orthosis provided the best immobilization of C1-C2 in limiting flexion and extension and 0-C1 in extension. The plastazote Philadelphia collar did not immobilize the cervical spine as well as the other orthoses. Like the polyethylene, the plastazote was significantly less effective than the SOMI or four-poster in restricting motion.

From review of the literature, it appears that splinting the cervical spine can offer temporary relief of pain and primarily serve as a reminder to patients to hold their necks in a neutral or slightly flexed position. As many types of cervical orthoses are currently being used, ranging from soft collars to more supportive orthoses, such as the SOMI brace, the basis for determining which collar is the most effective is based on the degree of immobilization required and the extent of disease activity. Other factors include the comfort of the collar and the ability of the patient to don and doff the collar or brace easily.

Summary

Splinting is of value during the acute phase of an arthritis problem; goals range from relief of pain and inflammation to improvement of function. Splints may be worn continuously in the very active phase of rheumatoid disease and used intermittently when symptoms improve. Several studies indicate there is no risk of permanent joint stiffness from either continuous or intermittent splinting.

Splinting for Prevention or Correction of Deformity

Few studies have objectively measured the effects of splinting for prevention or correction of deformity, so the role of splinting for these purposes remains controversial. In order to fully understand the role of corrective splinting, we will review the deformities and pathomechanics of the rheumatoid hand.

Deformity at the MCP Joint

Deformities occuring at the MCP joint of the hand are usually manifested by ulnar drift and palmar subluxation. Various authors attribute the following reasons for the development of ulnar drift.[31-34]

Recurring bouts of synovitis may cause stretching of the collateral ligaments and weakening of the supporting structures, later resulting in dislocation of the long extensor and flexor tendons. Secondly, pain and stretching of the joint capsule can cause muscle spasm and contracture of the ulnar intrinsic muscles. Thirdly, radial deviation deformities of the wrist which develop as a result of synovitis can result in the fingers developing ulnar drift to maintain alignment; this is referred to as the "zig-zag effect."

Some authors have recommended that splinting may be of value in the early phase of ulnar drift in order to provide optimal alignment of the MCP joints.[35-37] Czap[38] has stated that splinting may provide proper counterforces to restore balance to the hand structures, and Bennett[39] recommends the use of splints to allow motion in the normal planes, thereby blocking faulty planes and preventing instability and malalignment. Smith and associates[33] also recommend splinting to prevent deformity by altering the dynamic flexor forces. Although splinting may be of help in the early stage of MCP dysfunction, there is no objective evidence to substantiate this. However, there is objective evidence of the inability of splinting to correct existing deformity. In a study by Convery and associates, 51 patients with deformity were fitted with dynamic splints. The authors concluded that correction of existing deformity was not achieved and that the progression of deformity was not consistently prevented.[40] According to Flatt, many physicians feel that splinting has no place in the management of ulnar drift since this deformity is dynamically induced.[3]

The basic function of most splints in the treatment of ulnar drift is to stabilize the MCP joints so as to improve hand function. Several splints have been used in an attempt to control this deformity; however, none of these splints will correct joint dislocation.[3] Their purpose and basic design are similar.

Ulnar Deviation Splints

Goals

Maintain joint alignment
Control ulnar drift during activity
Improve function

Treatment Principles. These splints are usually made of low temperature, thermoplastic materials. (Figs. 8-11 to 8-13). They are sometimes difficult to mold comfortably and may be cumbersome. In addition, many patients complain that these splints are unsatisfactory because they partially limit flexion of the MCP joints, forcing grasp to occur at the distal portion of the digits.

Deformity at the Proximal Interphalangeal Joint

The swan neck deformity, which involves flexion of the MCP joint, hyperextension of the the proximal interphalangeal (PIP) joint, and flexion at the distal interphalangeal (DIP) joint, is another frequently encountered deformity in the rheumatoid hand. Although all swan neck deformities look alike, they vary in origin. Initial involvement may occur at the MCP, PIP, or DIP joint.

Flatt states that the most common cause of the swan neck deformity is tightness of the intrinsic musculature, which can occur initially as a result of chronic inflammation at the MCP joints.[3] A second type of involvement may

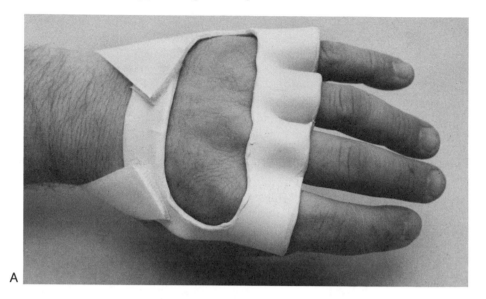

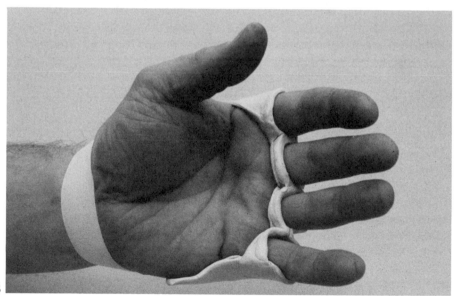

Fig. 8-11. (A,B) Quest-Cordery ulnar deviation splint provides abduction of the digits.

occur because of chronic synovitis at the PIP joints which stretches the volar plate.[1] Third, chronic inflammation at DIP joints may cause stretching or rupture at the insertion of the extensor tendon to the distal joint.[1]

Bennett has recommended the use of ring splints to overcome hyperextension of the PIP joints in the midstage of rheumatoid arthritis.[39] Although

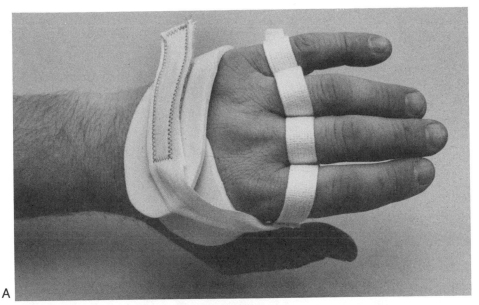

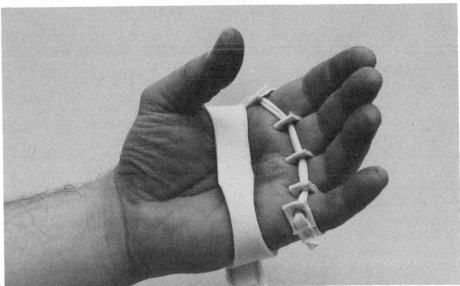

Fig. 8-12. (A,B)   Modified metacarpal ulnar drift (MUD) splint provides abduction of the digits.

the effectiveness of this type of splinting is unproven, informal reports suggest that this type of splint may contribute to tightening of the volar plate.[1]

The boutonnière deformity, characterized by flexion of the PIP joint and hyperextension at the DIP joint, has its origin at the PIP joint. This deformity occurs as a result of lengthening of the central slip of the extensor tendon and

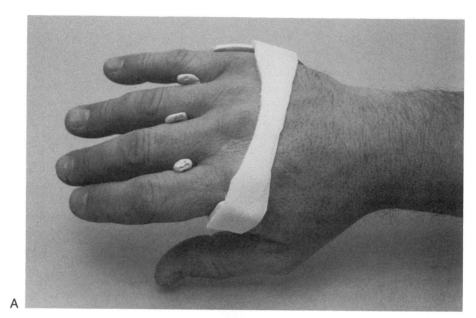

A

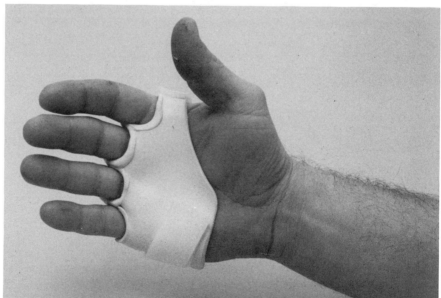

B

Fig. 8-13. (A,B) Ulnar deviation splint provides abduction of the digits.

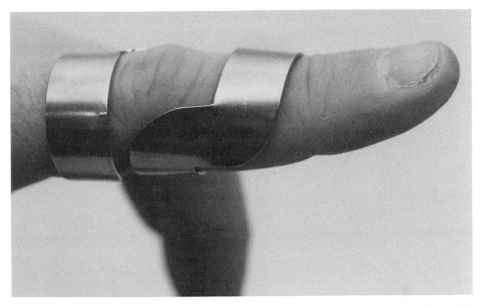

Fig. 8-14.   Ring splint for swan–neck deformity prohibits hyperextension of the PIP joint.

displacement of the lateral bands in a lateral, volar direction. Ring splinting has also been recommended in the early stages of this deformity, but again, its value is unproven.[39]

Ring Splints for Swan Neck Deformity

Goals

Limit hyperextension of the PIP joint
Improve function

Treatment Principles. Ring splints are commercially available or may be fabricated by using low temperature splinting materials. (Fig. 8-14). They should fit loosely to provide for easy donning and doffing, but should fit snugly enough to prevent slipping. When worn on adjacent fingers, they tend to catch, one on the other.

When swan neck deformity is due to intrinsic muscle tightness, Melvin recommends splinting with a wrist and MCP stabilization splint to counteract intrinsic tightness[16,18] (see Fig. 8-3).

Ring Splints for Boutonnière Deformity

Goal

Reduce contraction of the PIP Joint

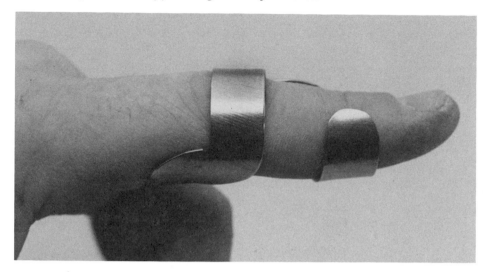

Fig. 8-15.   Ring splint for boutonniere deformity prohibits flexion of the PIP joint.

Treatment Principles. Ring splints are rarely used for the treatment of boutonniére deformity since most of these deformities in the early stage do not limit function. When 40° to 50° of extension at the PIP joint is lost, function is more severely hampered, but surgery is usually recommended at this stage to restore PIP joint extension by tightening the central slip and relocating the lateral bands (Fig. 8-15).

Deformity of the Thumb

Nalebuff has categorized thumb deformities from rheumatoid arthritis into four basic types. Type 1, the most common deformity, involves flexion of the MCP joint and hyperextension of the PIP joint. Type 2 deformity resembles the Type 1 deformity with the addition of CMC joint involvement. In Type 3 deformity, the PIP joint assumes a flexed position and the MCP joint is held in extension in association with CMC joint involvement. The fourth type of deformity involves CMC adduction and lateral deviation at the MCP joint.

Ring Splints for Thumb Hyperextension

Goals

Limit hyperextension of the PIP joint
Provide stability
Improve pinch prehension
Improve function

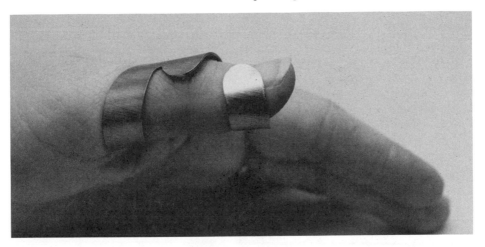

Fig. 8-16. Ring splint for thumb hyperextension prohibits hyperextension of the interphalangeal joint of the thumb.

Treatment Principles. Stability is most important for useful function of the thumb, and it is widely accepted that splinting can accomplish this goal. Although splinting will not alter the disease progression or correct the deformity of the rheumatoid thumb, it can be used as a temporary measure to improve function (Fig. 8-16). Ring splints made of metal or splints fabricated from thermoplastic low temperature materials may be used to stabilize the PIP or MCP joints of the thumb. Ring splints have a high patient acceptability and allow exposure of maximum skin surface for functional purposes.

Dynamic Splinting

Dynamic splinting for the hand has been recommended by Bunnell[41] and Flatt[3] as being effective in reducing flexion or extension contractures of MCPs and PIPs, particularly in postoperative care. Dynamic splints achieve their effect by the application of a gentle and persistent force to which scar tissue will yield. The tension for this type of splinting is achieved by rubber bands or springs, and frequent readjustment of the tension is necessary to prevent aggravation of joint pathology. Therefore, this type of splinting should only be used with patients who can be available for frequent monitoring of progress. This type of splinting should be discontinued within 3 weeks if significant progress is not noted by then (Figs. 8-17 to 8-23).

Summary

The value of the use of splints for prevention or correction of rheumatoid deformities remains unproven. However, dynamic splinting may be of great value as part of a preoperative or postoperative treatment program. A thorough

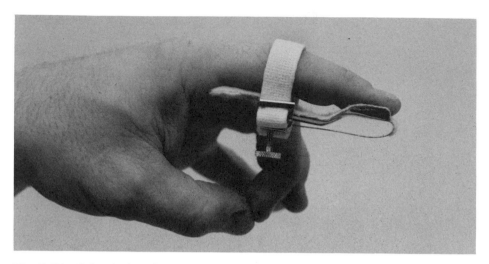

Fig. 8-17. Joint–jack splint provides dynamic extension to the proximal interphalangeal joint for flexion contractures of 30° or less.

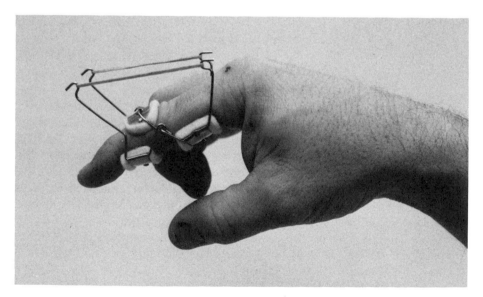

Fig. 8-18. Reverse finger knuckle bender provides dynamic extension to the proximal interphalangeal joint by rubber bands.

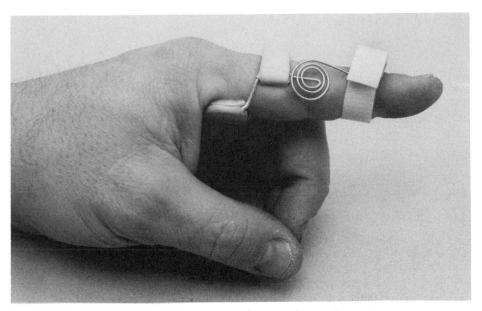

Fig. 8-19. Capener splint provides dynamic extension assist to the proximal interphalangeal joint with a three-point pressure system.

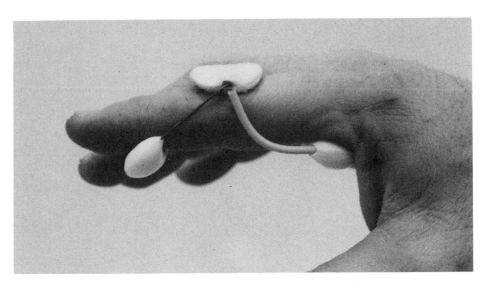

Fig. 8-20. LMB finger extension splint provides dynamic extension assist to the proximal interphalangeal joint by the use of wire cords to alter passive joint motion.

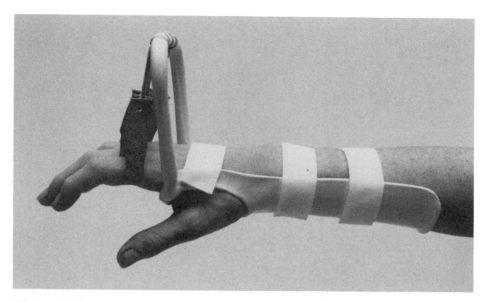

Fig. 8-21. Dynamic extension assist splint controls alignment of the fingers and assists metacarpophalangeal joint extension.

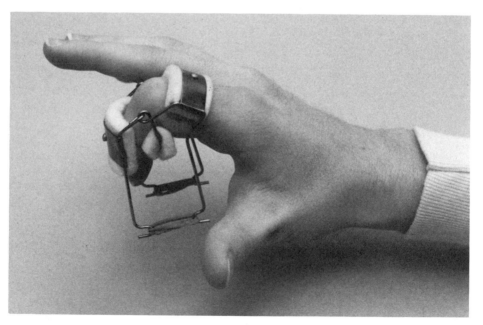

Fig. 8-22. Knuckle bender splint provides a flexion assist to the proximal interphalangeal joint.

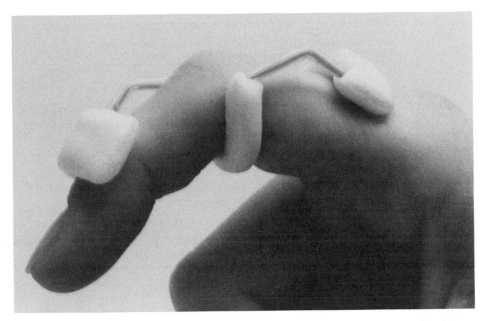

Fig. 8-23. LMB finger flexion splint provides a flexion assist to the proximal interphalangeal joint.

knowledge of the pathologic factors contributing to an existing problem is required in making decisions regarding indications for use of a particular splint.

Splinting for Improvement of Function

The use of splinting for improvement of function has been described by many authors[3,20,36] Flatt supports the use of splints as substitutes for loss of muscle power or as a protection for weakened muscles of the hand, and Melvin reports the use of wrist stabilization splints to eliminate pain, improve grasp and thereby improve hand function.[3,1]

For many patients, activities or job tasks may become easier when performed with the use of splints, as they can provide support for weakened structures and offer symptomatic pain relief. For example, patients who perform dexterous job tasks may find hand function is enhanced by the use of static wrist or thumb stabilization splints.

The therapist, who plays a key role in addressing the functions that enable a patient to carry out his daily activities, may be asked to make a visit on the job site or perform a simulated work assessment to determine the effects of splinting for improving a patient's job tasks. Adaptions and the utilization of splints in the work environment may be made with discussion and assistance from a patient's employer to enable some patients to continue employment.

Table 8-1. Splints Used to Improve Function

Volar resting splints	Static thumb splints
Static wrist splints	Ulnar deviation splints
Wrist splint with thumb attachment	Ring splints

Overall, the utilization of splinting to improve function is of proven efficacy. However, functional splints must be individually designed to fulfill specific needs.

Summary

Classification of splints for improvement of hand function is difficult, because most splints serve several functions. A variety of splints that can be used for relief of pain, relief of inflammation and improvement of joint stability will serve also to improve hand function (Table 8-1).

Fabrication Considerations

There are many types of splinting materials currently on the market, ranging from high temperature materials such as Kydex and Nyloplex to low temperature materials such as Orthoplast and Plastazote. The choice of splinting material depends largely on the skill of the fabricator. Table 8-2 lists other factors to be considered when choosing splinting materials. For a more thorough listing of splinting materials, refer to the following sources by Maude Malick: "Manual on Static Hand Splinting"[42] and "Manual on Dynamic Hand Splinting with Thermoplastic Materials."[43]

High temperature materials must be formed over a positive mold, whereas low temperature materials can be formed directly on the patient. Advantages of high temperature materials are that they can be exposed to heat without losing shape and they are rigid and durable. The low temperature materials will deform when exposed to heat (e.g., leaving a splint on a radiator or in the hot sun) and generally are not as durable. Nevertheless, most therapists seem to favor the low temperature materials because of their ease of fabrication and cosmetic acceptability.

To facilitate effectiveness with a splinting program, certain questions should be considered:

Does the splint meet the goals of the therapist and the patient?
Does the splint limit function?
Does the splint fit?

Splints should be designed so that they can be put on and removed without assistance, and they should fit comfortably to encourage compliance by the

Table 8-2. Aspects to Consider When Choosing Splinting Material

Patient comfort or allergies	Cleaning ability
Ability of patient to don and doff splint	Cost of splinting material
Patient's occupation	Skill of fabricator
Cosmetic acceptability	Ease and rapidity of fabrication
Weight of splint	Ease of adjustment

patient. No matter how effective or cleverly designed a splint may be, if it is uncomfortable or causes limitations in function, its use will be of short duration (Table 8-2).

Educating the Patient Regarding Splints

In order to achieve the goals of the splinting program, the patient should be given specific guidelines for splint wear and care. Effective education is essential so that patients may avoid secondary problems resulting from incorrect splint usage. Before a splint is issued, the patient should understand and agree with the goals of splinting and its relationship with the overall program. In addition, instructions to the patient should be specific regarding when the splint should be worn and what exercises should be performed in conjunction with the splinting program. Written instructions should be given to the patient to avoid confusion. The patient should also be asked to demonstrate unassisted donning and doffing of the splint to make sure all instructions are correctly understood. On return visits to the therapist, a worn and dirty splint is a good sign that the patient has been compliant with wearing the splint while a clean one is a flag for re-evaluation of this portion of the treatment program. Other educational guidelines are listed in Table 8-3.

Table 8-3. Instructions for Splint Wear and Care

Purpose of splint	Proper fit
Wearing schedule	Cleaning of splint
Splint adjustments	Exercise program

JOINT PROTECTION PRINCIPLES

A rationale for joint protection training was first described by Cordery in 1965.[44] Joint protection training has since become an integral component of a comprehensive program for the rheumatic disease patient. Training in joint protection techniques enables the arthritis patient with early disease to maintain maximum levels of function while reducing pain and stress to involved joints. However, controversy continues to exist over the value of the activity of joint protection for prevention of deformity and its use during periods of disease remission, because good controlled studies have not been done. The need for research in this area is strongly evident.

There are numerous methods for teaching joint protection techniques, and over the years written materials and audiovisual presentations have been developed to assist in this phase of patient education. One effective method, developed by Gruen and Wingert, is based on the use of "the four Ps": pacing, planning, priorities, and positioning. These four basic principles, which are described below, may be effective for conserving energy and protecting joints. Other guidelines for joint protection training may be found in publications by Cordery,[44] Melvin,[1,16] and the Arthritis Clearinghouse.[47]

Pacing

Effective pacing allows patients with rheumatoid arthritis to accomplish more while protecting inflamed joints. Convincing patients that the principles of pacing should be followed regardless of the intensity of disease activity is oftentimes a difficult task. On "bad days," patients tend to do too little and on "good days," they tend to overdo.

Encouraging patients to evaluate the effectiveness of pacing is sometimes helpful. For example, suggesting that patients ask such questions as "Did I have less pain or stiffness after pacing myself yesterday?" or "When I didn't pace myself, did I feel tired or stiff? " enables patients to judge the benefits of pacing. Most patients eventually realize that by pacing themselves, especially on the "good days," they will note less pain and stiffness and are than motivated to continue to follow pacing principles.

Principles for Pacing

Take frequent rest breaks throughout the day.
Take breaks during activities before you begin to feel tired.
On good days, pace your work so you will feel less tired at the end of the day.
On a structured job, utilize lunch and coffee breaks for rest periods.

Planning

Instructing patients to plan their activities on a daily and weekly basis will enable them to conserve energy and accomplish more in the long run. This principle can best be understood by teaching patients to plan small amounts of work each day and to alternate heavier and lighter tasks. This will enable them to conserve energy and alleviate stress to involved joints. Encourage patients to use a calendar to plan their week, spacing out their activities, as opposed to trying to accomplish all of their work on 1 or 2 days.

Principles for Planning

Plan small amounts of work each day; don't overdo.
Follow a heavy task with a less demanding task.

Priorities

Effective planning requires the establishment of priorities. Patients should list activities in order of importance. Prioritizing tasks will enable patients to save energy in certain areas and expend it in others. For example, a homemaker who tires easily may decide to postpone doing the laundry so that she can go out to dinner with her family that evening. She could try to do everything, but she might end up being too tired to enjoy the dinner. For some patients, setting priorities will require making changes in not only daily routines, but also eliminating certain activities of lesser importance.

Principles for Setting Priorities

Make a list of chores in order of importance.
If you feel tired or in pain, postpone certain activities until another day.

Positioning

The principles of positioning allow patients to protect their joints and to avoid pain and stress. Positioning also reduces fatigue. For example, joint stress and fatigue may occur by staying in one position for long periods of time or by using the smaller joints of the hand to perform heavy tasks.

It is important to educate patients to change positions frequently and to position their joints in ways that avoid stress and the potential for deformity. This is accomplished by teaching patients specific techniques (e.g., carrying a purse on the elbow as opposed to the fingers) or recommending the use of assistive devices to perform self-care and household tasks.

Principles for Positioning

Use the stronger or larger joints when performing heavy tasks.
Use each joint in its most stable and anatomic plane to reduce potential for deformity.
Change positions frequently.
Use assistive devices to prevent joint stress.

Patient Compliance

Informal reports on rates of patient compliance with prescribed joint protection programs suggest that enhancing patient cooperation presents a critical challenge. Compliance is affected by such factors as the ability of the patient to make changes in lifestyle or the ability to deal with reduced function or loss of independence. Emotional responses such as anger, denial, or guilt are common.

For some patients, incorporating the principles of joint protection may mean making changes in their daily routine or eliminating certain tasks and relying on friends or family members to help. This may cause some patients to experience guilt because they feel they are unable to fulfill their customary roles as family members. For example, homemakers often feel that they are depriving their children or husband if the family must perform some of the household duties; this is especially true for certain cultural or ethnic groups. Others may attempt to deny their disease or to disguise their disabilities by trying to do everything on their own so others will not think them lazy. The ability to deal with issues such as these secondarily affects compliance with joint protection training.

There is evidence to suggest that the planning, type, and timing of educational materials are important factors in influencing behavioral changes and compliance.[48] There are certain techniques that may be helpful in facilitating patients' understanding and follow-through with joint–protection training. During initial evaluation, the patient's lifestyle should be reviewed; an open discussion of activities should be encouraged, emphasizing those that are difficult or cause pain. The therapist should have a thorough understanding of the depth of the patient's knowledge of the disease and of expectations regarding the treatment program. This understanding is needed to assist the therapist in determining the need for specialized treatments. The educational process becomes easier once these items are clarified.

Instructions to the patient should be simple and easy to understand, and written material should supplement verbal instructions. Although instructions should be specific, patients should also be given general guidelines for when and how they can change their joint protection programs.[18] For example, patients may be instructed to utilize joint protection techniques when performing an activity that would cause pain in the presence of joint inflammation. However, instruction for making changes in this program when symptoms of inflammation subside should also be given. This type of educational approach allows the patient to be actively involved in the treatment program and makes him responsible for making adjustments as the disease process varies. Patients should also be taught to evaluate the effectiveness of treatment. Teaching patients to ask such questions as, "Do I have less pain or stiffness after pacing myself?" will allow them to judge the benefits of utilizing joint protection techniques.

Patients should be asked to demonstrate certain joint protection techniques and to state when the principles of joint protection should be applied. For example, have a patient demonstrate opening a jar the routine way and then demonstrate opening a jar using joint protection principles. This permits the therapist to evaluate the patient's understanding of the program.

Goal setting with the patient and family members is another effective method for enlisting the patient's involvement. This is accomplished by setting goals with the patient and then asking how he intends to meet these goals. At the next visit, the goals from the previous session should be reviewed and any difficulties with compliance should be discussed in a nonjudgmental fashion.

Instructing patients in a group setting tends to provide reinforcement. Group sessions allow patients to openly discuss their difficulties in meeting goals and permits sharing, suggestions, and solutions to common problems in making lifestyle changes.

Although patient education is often a difficult area for both patient and therapist, the utilization of the above principles may avoid patient confusion and assist in enhancing levels of compliance with prescribed joint protection programs. For more information, please refer to the literature on patient education.

Summary

The value of joint protection training lies in its effectiveness in enabling patients to continue performing their daily activities while conserving their energy and reducing pain and joint stress. It is important that joint protection programs be individualized to each patient's specific needs. Teaching patients to monitor the signs and symptoms of arthritic disease will enable them to determine when joint protection principles should be incorporated into their daily activities.

REFERENCES

1. Melvin JL: Rheumatic Disease: Occupational Therapy and Rehabilitation. FA Davis, Philadelphia, 1977
2. Swanson AB, Coleman JD: Corrective bracing needs of the rheumatoid arthritic wrist. Am Occup Ther 20:38, 1966
3. Flatt A: Care of the Arthritic Hand. 4th ed. CV Mosby, St. Louis, 1983
4. Overton J, Wolcott LE: The role of splints in the prevention of deformity in the rheumatoid hand and wrist. Missouri Med 63:423, 1966
5. Rotstein J: Use of splints in conservative management of acutely inflamed joints in rheumatoid arthritis. Arch Phys Med 46:198, 1965
6. Salvanelli M: Functional wrist splint for patients with rheumatoid arthritis. Phys Ther 44:743, 1964
7. Shalit IS, Decker JL: Silicone foam resting splints for rheumatoid arthritis. Lancet 1:142, 1965
8. VanBrocklin JD: Splinting the rheumatoid hand. Arch Phys Med 47:262, 1966

9. Partridge RE, Duthie JJ: Controlled trial of the effect of complete immobilization of the joints in rheumatoid arthritis. Ann Rheum Dis 22:91, 1963

10. Gault SJ, Spyker MJ: Beneficial effect of immobilization of joints in rheumatoid and related arthritides: A splint study using sequential analysis. Arthritis Rheum 12:34, 1969

11. Nicholas JJ, Ziegler G: Cylinder splints: Their use in the treatment of arthritis of the knee. Arch Phys Med Rehabil 58:264, 1977

12. Biddulph SL: The effect of the Futuro wrist brace in painful conditions of the wrists. S Afr Med J 60:389, 1981

13. Zoeckler AA, Nicholas JJ: Prenyl hand splint for rheumatoid arthritis. Phys Ther 49:377, 1969

14. Harris R, Copp EP: Immobilization of the knee joint in rheumatoid arthritis. Ann Rheum Dis 21:353, 1962

15. Swezey RL: Arthritis: Rational Therapy and Rehabilitation. WB Saunders, Philadelphia, 1978

16. Melvin JL: Rheumatic Disease: Occupational Therapy and Rehabilitation. 2nd ed. FA Davis, Philadelphia, 1982

17. Fess EE, Gettle KS, Strickland JW: Hand Splinting—Principles and Methods. CV Mosby, St. Louis, 1981

18. Riggs GE, Gall EP: Rheumatic Disease: Rehabilitation and Management. Butterworth (Publishers), Boston, 1984

19. Feinberg J, Brandt K: Use of resting splints by patients with rheumatoid arthritis. Am J Occup Ther 35:173, 1981

20. Gumpel JM, Cannon S: A cross-over comparison of ready-made fabric wrist splints in rheumatoid arthritis. Rheumatol Rehab 20:113, 1981

21. Ehrlich GE: Total Management of the Arthritic Patient. JB Lippincott, Philadelphia, 1973

22. Hunter JM, Schneider LH, Mackin EJ, Bell J: Rehabilitation of the Hand. CV Mosby, St. Louis, 1978

23. Askari A, Moskowitz RW, Ryan C: Stretch gloves: Study of objective and subjective effectiveness in arthritis of the hands. Arthritis Rheum 17:263, 1974

24. Ehrlich GE, DePiero AM: Stretch gloves: Nocturnal use to ameliorate morning stiffness in arthritic hands. Arch Phys Med Rehab 52:479, 1971

25. Culic DD, Battaglia MC, Wichman C, Schmid FR: Efficacy of compression gloves in rheumatoid arthritis. Am J Phys Med 58:278, 1979

26. Swezey RL, Speigel TM, Cretin S, Clements P: Arthritic hand response to pressure gradient gloves. Arch Phys Med Rehab 60:375, 1979

27. McKnight PT, Schomberg FL: Air pressure splint effects on hand symptoms of patients with rheumatoid arthritis. Arch Phys Med Rehab 63:560, 1982

28. Colachis SC, Strohm BR, Ganter EL: Cervical spine motion in normal women: Radiographic study of effect of cervical collars. Arch Phys Med Rehab 54:161, 1973

29. Hartman JT, Palumbo F, Hill BJ: Cineradiography of braced normal cervical spine: Comparative study of five commonly used cervical orthoses. Clin Orthop 109:97, 1975

30. Fisher SV, Bowar JF, Awad EA, Gullickson G: Cervical orthoses effect on cervical spine motion: Roentgenographic and goniometric method of study. Arch Phys Med Rehab 58:109, 1977

31. Swezey RL: Dynamic factors in deformity of the rheumatoid arthritic hand. Bull Rheum Dis 22:649, 1971–1972

32. English C, Nalebuff EA: Understanding the arthritic hand. Am J Occup Ther 25:352, 1971

33. Smith EM, Juvinall RC, Bender LF, Pearson JR: Role of the finger flexors in rheumatoid deformities of the metacarpophalangeal joints. Arthritis Rheum 7:467, 1964
34. Swanson AB, Swanson GD: Pathogenesis and pathomechanics of rheumatoid deformities in the hand and wrist. Orthop Clin N Am 4:1039, 1973
35. Spelbring LM: Splinting the arthritic hand. Am J Occup Ther 20:40, 1966
36. Quest IM, Cordery J: A functional ulnar deformity cuff for the rheumatoid deformity. AJOT 25:32, 1971
37. Houchin R, Cheshire L: Splintage for ulnar deviation. Am J Occup Ther 21:9, 1971
38. Czap L: Orthotic management of the rheumatoid hand. South Med J 59:115, 1966
39. Bennett RL: Orthotic devices to prevent deformities of the hand in rheumatoid arthritis. Arthritis Rheum 85:1006, 1965
40. Convery FR, Conaty JP, Nickel VL: Dynamic splinting of the rheumatoid hand. Orthotics and Prosthetics 21:249, 1967
41. Bunnell S: Surgery of the Hand. 3rd ed. JB Lippincott, Philadelphia, 1956
42. Malick MH: Manual on static hand splinting. Harmarville Rehabilitation Center, Pittsburgh, 1973
43. Malick MH: Manual on dynamic hand splinting with thermoplastic materials. Harmarville Rehabilitation Center, Pittsburgh, 1974
44. Cordery JC: Joint protection, a responsibility of the occupational therapist. Am J Occup Ther 19:285, 1965
45. Gruen H, Wingert B: Joint protection and energy conservation for the early rheumatoid arthritis patient (slide/tape). Graphics Plus Associates, Pittsburgh, 1976
46. Gruen H, Medsger T, White J: Joint protection training for the patient with early rheumatoid arthritis. Documenta Geigy Ciba-Geigy Limited, Switzerland, 1980
47. Arthritis Information Clearinghouse, PO Box 9782, Arlington, VA 22209
48. Gerber LH: Principles and their application in the rehabilitation of patients with rheumatoid disease. p. 1849. In Kelley WN, Harris ED, Ruddy S, Sledge CB (eds): Textbook of Rheumatology, WB Saunders, Philadelphia, 1981

9 | Physical Therapy Management of Juvenile Arthritis

Lenora W. Barnes

This chapter contains a brief description of the four connective tissue diseases most commonly seen by the therapist concerned with pediatric rheumatology: juvenile rheumtoid arthritis (JRA), juvenile ankylosing spondylitis (JAS), dermatomyositis, and scleroderma. Of these, JRA is by far the most recognized and prevalent, estimated at 135,000 to 200,000 children in the United States alone. The frequency of JAS may exceed this but because it is frequently not recognized in childhood, reliable estimates are not available.[1] Dermatomyositis and scleroderma are relatively rare diseases but present special problems for the therapist.

Systemic lupus erythematosis (SLE) occurs in children somewhat more frequently than dermatomyositis and scleroderma. These children may occasionally have muscle or joint pain and decreased range of motion. In long term cases an aseptic necrosis may develop in a joint requiring exercise to maintain range of motion and, if a weight bearing joint is involved, crutches or canes to provide support. A program of exercise may aid in preventing osteoporosis from long-term steroid treatment.

Specific details of physical therapy evaluation and treatment are discussed under each disease. Some general concepts of treatment for children with rheumatologic diseases and designing a home program for them are found under physical therapy treatment of JRA later in this chapter.

JUVENILE RHEUMATOID ARTHRITIS

The classic modern description of both acute and chronic JRA was made in 1896 by George Frederick Still, an English pediatrician. He mentioned the increased frequency in girls, the tendency to early contractures and muscle atrophy, and the high incidence of cervical spine disease. The acute systemic onset of JRA with inflammation of joints, splenomegaly, hepatomegaly, fever, pleuritis, pericarditis, anemia and growth retardation is still called Still's disease.

Diagnosis

The diagnosis of JRA has been aided by the recognition of three types of onset: systemic, polyarticular, and pauciarticular. The diagnosis is made by exclusion of other possible causes of joint inflammation such as infection, neoplasm, trauma, blood disease, and allergy, and by time. Persistent joint disease must be present for at least 6 weeks, manifested by swelling or limitation of motion with heat, pain, or tenderness. Children with systemic onset may have fever, rash, hepato- and splenomegaly, pericarditis, and other general symptoms of inflammation with little or no joint manifestation. They must, however, exhibit the required signs of arthritis for a definite diagnosis to be made.[2]

Laboratory tests are frequently not helpful in diagnosis. Fifteen percent of children with JRA will have a positive rheumatoid factor, not enough to be a reliable diagnostic test. The erythrosedimentation rate, white blood cell count, and differential may all be elevated, but they are only general indicators of inflammation. It is important to test for the presence of antinuclear antibody (ANA) because of the increased risk of chronic uveitis when it is positive. JRA can also overlap with systemic lupus erythematosis in children, and a change from negative to positive ANA may signal this.[3]

Age of onset peaks at about 2 years with another lower peak at 9 years.[4] Grouping all types of onset together the female to male ratio is 2:1.

Etiology is unknown. Potential causative factors under investigation include infection, autoimmunity, trauma, psychological stress, and heredity.[5,6]

Types of Onset (Table 9-1)

Systemic

The most striking symptom of systemic onset is a daily spiking fever which then returns to normal. It can occur at any time but is usual in the late afternoon. The rash of JRA may occur with the fever, though it can occur alone (Fig. 9-1). It is a pink, macular eruption of circumscribed lesions usually found on the

Table 9-1. Types of Onset of JRA

	Polyarthritis	Oligoarthritis	Systemic Disease
Percent of cases	50%	40%	10%
Sex (F:M)	2:1	2:1	1:1
Age of onset	Through childhood Peak at 2 years	Early childhood Peak at 2 years	Through childhood No peak
Joints	5 or more	4 or fewer	Variable
Systemic features	Variable	None	Fever, rash, leukocytosis, organomegaly
Chronic uveitis	5%	20%	None
Rheumatoid nodules	10%	Rare	Rare
Rheumatoid factors	15% (age-related)	Rare	Rare
Antinuclear antibodies	40%	70% (with uveitis)	15%
HLA-B27	8%	12%	8%
Prognosis	Good	Excellent (except eyes)	Moderately good

(Cassidy JT (ed): Textbook of Pediatric Rheumatology. p. 179. John Wiley & Sons, New York, 1982.)

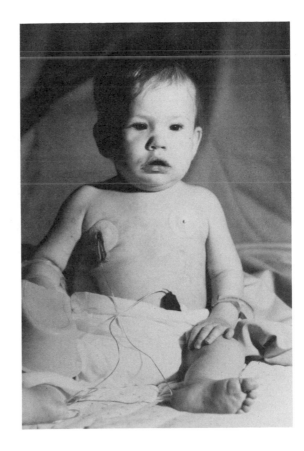

Fig. 9-1. TH diagnosed at 10 months with systemic onset of JRA, including fevers, hepatosplenomegaly, and pericarditis. Note rash of JRA on her abdomen and her general distressed appearance. Passive joint range of motion remained within normal limits but she would not attempt to stand. (Photo courtesy of David Merzel, MD, Department of Pediatric Rheumatology, University of Michigan.)

trunk, thighs, and upper arms. It comes and goes at irregular intervals and is rarely pruritic. These children usually have hepato- and splenomegaly as described by Still, and may have pericarditis. They are usually quite ill during the fever spikes, but may be well otherwise. The systemic symptoms may be present long before they have any arthritic complaints, but arthritis must be present to make a definite diagnosis.[5-7]

Systemic onset occurs in about 10 percent of the total cases of JRA. Fifty percent of the children with this onset will recover almost completely. The other 50 percent will go on to have polyarticular disease with moderate to severe disability.[7] This group is most at risk for life-threatening complications,[6] and for general growth retardation.[8]

Polyarticular

A child must have arthritis in five or more joints to be classified as polyarticular. These children may have systemic symptoms but usually not as acutely as in that type of onset. The knees, wrists, and ankles are most commonly involved joints. (Fig. 9-2). The small joints are more often involved than they are in pauciarticular onset. Morning stiffness is common. Bony growth deformities include early maturation of epiphyses with resultant small bones. In more severe cases this is evidenced by micrognathia, giving a distinct facies.[5-7]

About 50 percent of all children with JRA present with polyarticular onset. A satisfactory prognosis can be expected in most of the children. However, there is a group whose disease is characterized by polyarthritic disease, prominent systemic manifestations, articular erosions, long duration of active disease, rheumatoid factor positivity, and rheumatoid nodules who are at risk for an unsatisfactory outcome.[6]

Pauciarticular

Approximately 40 percent of the total cases of JRA involve four or less joints and are classified as pauciarticular disease. (Fig. 9-3). One quarter of the children who present with pauciarticular onset will go on to further joint involvement and become polyarticular. The knee is the most commonly involved joint, followed by the wrist, hip, and elbow. If only one joint is involved, it is the knee in 75 percent of cases.[6] These children rarely have systemic symptoms and may seem to ignore their joint disease. Occasionally with an acutely swollen knee or ankle the child will stop walking. In such cases there should be immediate medical intervention.

The child with pauciarticular arthritis who has a positive ANA is at risk for development of chronic uveitis, an inflammation of the eye. Recognition, treatment, and prognosis have improved for this condition, but there is still

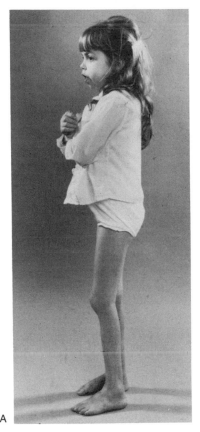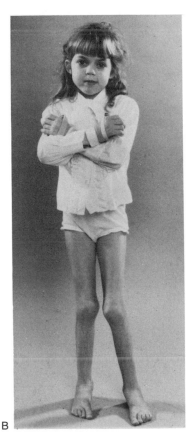

A   B

Fig. 9-2. (A,B) MH had onset of polyarticular arthritis at 18 months and has continued to have severe disease that has not responded well to antiinflammatory medication. She carries out a daily program of exercise at home with her parents and with a school therapist, and has remained ambulatory in spite of hip and knee involvement. Note the flexed right great toe, the valgus of the lower leg, internal rotation of the hips, and increased lordosis secondary to hip flexion contractures. She is wearing resting wrist orthoses. (Photo courtesy of Donita B Sullivan, MD, Department of Pediatric Rheumatology, University of Michigan.)

risk of blindness. Visual loss can develop before objective symptoms can be seen in routine exam. The only method of early detection is by a slit-lamp exam performed by an opthalmologist. All children with JRA are at risk for chronic uveitis and should have regular slit-lamp exams with the pauciarticular ANA positive child having more frequent checks.[5,6,9]

Knee or ankle involvement with accompanying growth disturbance of the long bones can lead to a leg–length discrepancy. Early detection and treatment will minimize secondary complications such as flexion contractures and scoliosis.

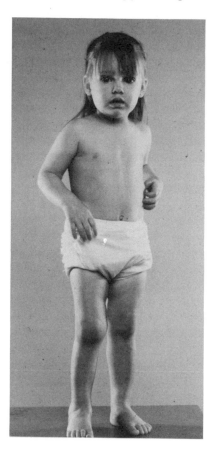

Fig. 9-3. KM at 28 months. She presented at 20 months with a swollen right knee and ankle. These have continued to be the only joints involved. She has a half inch leg–length discrepancy which is partially corrected with a quarter inch lift on the left shoe. Note the typical posture of the longer right lower extremity: flexed, abducted, and externally rotated. (Photo courtesy of Carol G Ragsdale, MD, Department of Pediatric Rheumatology, University of Michigan.)

Radiologic Joint Changes

The earliest radiologic signs in JRA are soft tissue swelling and osteoporosis. In pauciarticular disease these may be the only signs that develop. In polyarticular and systemic JRA periosteal new bone is sometimes laid down. This gives the metacarpals a characteristic thickened appearance. There is early maturation of the epiphyseal ossification centers and enlargement of the epiphyses.[6] This does not occur in pauciarticular disease in spite of intense local inflammation.

Later in the course of the disease growth arrest lines may appear. Cartilage and bone destruction lead to ankylosis and subluxation. Ankylosis occurs more promptly in JRA than in adult RA. Fusion of the carpal and tarsal bones is common and is frequently associated with cervical spine fusion, usually of C2 and C3.[6,10] Subluxation occurs in both small and large joints. It is a possible complication of hip involvement. The wrist is also a common site of subluxation. Atlantoaxial subluxation in the cervical spine must be carefully assessed for possible neurologic signs.

Epiphyseal and vertebral compression fractures are seen in severe, long-term disease, after long immobilizations, and especially where there has been extended treatment with corticosteroids.[6,11]

Growth Deformities

Isdale has termed growth deformities the main difference between JRA and RA.[12] Overgrowth of the long bones at the affected joints occurs in one half of the children with pauciarticular onset. This can lead to a leg–length discrepancy even when there is bilateral disease. There is undergrowth of the small round and tubular bones such as the carpal and tarsal bones. In the wrist this results in intercarpal joint space narrowing, changes in carpal bone shape, and bony fusion.[10] Early epiphyseal closure occurs in systemic onset and results in decreased size relative to the unaffected bones. A striking example being the micrognathia seen in children with long standing disease of early onset. These disturbances occur in polyarticular disease also, but early epiphyseal maturation is not common.[6,8,13]

Prognosis

Seventy to 90 percent of children with JRA recover with no serious disability. Ten percent have severe functional disability as they reach adulthood.[5,6] In an English study 15 years after onset of disease 85 percent of those children who were past school age were employed.[14] In a study of 121 young adults 18 years or older their status compared well to their unaffected siblings with 70 percent being either full time employees or students.[15] In light of the guardedly optimistic outlook for children with JRA, prevention of joint deformity takes on great importance.

Contrasts with Adult Rheumatoid Arthritis

JRA differs from adult rheumatoid arthritis in several ways. There is more frequent involvement of large joints rather than small. The patterns of common joint deformities vary in JRA (i.e., ulnar deviation at the wrist with radial deviation of the fingers). Muscle contracture and atrophy occur early while destruction of articular surfaces is a late occurrence. Some patients will have only systemic symptoms while others may have arthritis in only a few joints. Disturbances of growth patterns occur secondary to the inflammation of the disease, and naturally influence children while they are not a concern in adults. Cervical spine disease occurs early and without other spinal involvement. Children with arthritis are at risk for the development of potentially blinding chronic uveitis. It is important to remember that most children with JRA have the potential to be free of active arthritis by the time they are young adults.[5,6,16]

Treatment

The goals of treatment for children with connective tissue disease are to control the inflammatory process; to prevent deformity and maximize function; and to support and promote a sound psychosocial development. These goals can best be achieved by a multidisciplinary team. Headed by a pediatric rheumatologist, it should include a physical therapist, occupational therapist, social worker, and nurse. Orthopedists, physiatrists, and orthotists are frequently consulted. Regular eye exams by an opthalmologist are mandatory. Because of the early age of onset, it is very important that the entire team be familiar with normal growth and development and accomplishment of milestones, the object being to produce an age–related treatment plan.[17]

Drug Therapy

Aspirin.   Aspirin (acetylsalicyclic acid, ASA) is the drug of choice in combating the inflammation in arthritic joints. It is the safest of the drugs available for treatment of children with arthritis. Its side effects are well known and are usually the most easily controlled.

The optimum dose in children is that which will give a serum ASA level of 20 to 30 mg/dl. This is approximately 100 mg/kg of body weight. While the exact dosage required is being established, some children may show signs of aspirin toxicity. If this occurs, the usual procedure is stop aspirin for 24 hours, force fluids, and then restart the aspirin at a lower dosage.[7]

Determining toxicity is more difficult in the child than in the adult. Adults will complain at the early sign of tinnitus. Children do not complain, although they may pull at their ears.[18] The most reliable signs in children are hyperpnea, drowsiness, and lethargy. Parents are instructed to observe the rate and depth of their child's breathing when resting or asleep. Parents are aware of the frequency of aspirin poisoning in childhood and are sometimes reluctant to give the child the required dosage. They must be made aware that the aspirin is not just for the relief of pain but must be given regularly to achieve an anti-inflammatory effect. If they are well instructed in the signs of toxicity, they should feel comfortable in administering the amount required.

A common side effect of aspirin is gastrointestinal disturbance, which may rarely lead to ulcers. The physician emphasizes to the parents that the aspirin must be given with meals or a snack containing milk. This is usually enough to prevent gastric irritation. The food raises the pH of stomach contents and the salicylates penetrate the mucosal lining less easily. There is also more rapid passage into the intestine and therefore less irritation.[18]

Nonsteroidal Anti-inflammatory Drugs.   In the last several years many of these drugs have been introduced and are available for use in adults. At the present time only naproxen and tolmetin are approved by the United States Food and Drug Administration for use in children.

Gold.   Gold salts have been used in the treatment of arthritis in both adults and children since the 1920s. It is one of the few drugs that can cause a remission in arthritis. In children it is considered when there has not been a good response, when progression of disease is seen in spite of therapeutic doses of aspirin for 6 months, or when the child is corticosteroid dependent. Water soluble gold salts are given by intermuscular injection. At first they are given weekly and after a certain dosage level is attained, they are gradually spaced out. If there is a good response to the treatment, it is continued indefinitely.[6,19,20]

Toxic side effects include renal or hepatic damage, dermatitis, various abnormalities of blood cell counts, and gastrointestinal symptoms. Studies documenting normal blood, liver, and kidney function must be performed before gold is instituted and continue to be monitored during its use. Approximately 25 percent of the children started on gold will have their treatment terminated because of toxic reactions.[5]

There must be a commitment to the treatment on the part of the child, the parents, and an available physician who is familiar with gold therapy and its potentially serious side effects if it is to be used.[7] If these conditions cannot be met, gold should not be prescribed.

Corticosteroids. Steroids are used reluctantly by most physicians. They are reserved for cases of severe or life-threatening JRA, such as the child with pericarditis or other severe systemic disease or the child with acute uveitis which has not responded to local steroid therapy.[6,7,21]

The side effects include osteoporosis, which can lead to collapsed vertebrae; glaucoma; cataracts; psychosis; peptic ulceration; and hypertension. Since JRA can of itself result in diminished skeletal growth, the additional stunting effect of steroids can produce significant loss of stature.[22]

Because of the serious potential side effects, when steroids must be used, they are tapered as soon as possible. However, their use results in a dampening of the body's own adrenocortical system. Therefore, the taper must be very careful to avoid an acute adrenal insufficiency. After each cut in dosage, the child may experience a few days of increased pain and stiffness until the body readjusts its adrenal output.[23] Parents should be aware of this so they will not interpret the child's discomfort as a flare of the arthritis.

Systemic steroids suppress the body's response to inflammation and so reduce fever, rash, and joint effusion. Their use will not limit or change the course of the disease and may increase the chance of complications.[22,23] Medical emergencies or surgeries will require that a higher dose be reinstituted.[5,22]

Physical Therapy Evaluation

In all types of JRA, physical therapy is most associated with the second goal of treatment—prevention of deformity. Modalities, exercise, and activities are used to maintain range of motion and strength. The specific program designed for each child is based, of course, on a careful evaluation of that child.

Observation

Much can be learned by observing the child and parents as they come into the clinic. Facial expression and ease of movement are indicators of the child's present status. Is the parent carrying the child? Any difficulty observed in walking and getting on the examining table or mat or in and out of a chair should be noted. Can the child remove his or her own clothes? Do the parents allow this?

Arthritic enlargement of joints may be quite visible when the involved joints are the knee, ankle, wrist, or fingers. The elbow or shoulder require closer examination, and cervical spine or hip swelling may be almost impossible to detect. Warmth of the joints is determined manually by comparing the temperature of the joint to another uninvolved joint or to an adjacent area of the body. Tenderness may be elicited as the therapist goes through the range of motion evaluation or by specifically palpating around involved joints. There is often swelling without tenderness but most young children complain less of pain than adults[24] or have difficulty localizing it to specific joints. Thus it is important to observe the child's reaction to movement during the evaluation.

Teenagers may report more pain because of increased understanding of JRA and the joint pathology involved. More information may be gained from the young child by asking about "feelings" in the joint rather than about pain.[25]

Muscle Testing

Detailed muscle tests are not usually required for JRA but a gross examination of general strength should be done from time to time. With very young children, their ability to go up and down stairs, get up from the floor, and walk on heels or tiptoes may give a better assessment of functional strength than trying to gain their cooperation in a formal muscle test.

Self-splinting and abnormal use of joints may lead quite quickly to muscle atrophy, first seen in extensors and later in flexors.[6] Atrophy is easily seen in quadriceps medius and gastrocnemius when there is lower extremity involvement. Circumference should be recorded, measured at the fullest part of calf and thigh. In the ambulatory child lower extremity muscles retain near normal strength while shoulder girdle and upper extremity muscle groups may exhibit disuse atrophy. Hand strength can decrease when there is wrist involvement. In such cases specific muscle strength and/or grip strength should be measured.

Goniometry

Range of motion is measured using an appropriately-sized goniometer. Measurements are helpful in monitoring the course of disease, as part of baseline studies before initiation of new medication and for evaluating the effectiveness of the home exercise program.

Passive range of motion will usually provide a more reliable record with young children but a record of active range may also be kept. It is important to include the angle of the resting position of the hand if there is ulnar deviation of the wrist, and that of the fingers where radial deviation is most common. When measuring cervical spine ranges, remember to eliminate trunk movement. Knee flexion is most precisely measured in the prone position, but in children who have difficulty assuming this position, repetitive measures done in the supine position will indicate progression. End range limitation of knee flexion may be expressed as inches between heel and buttock. Children should be able to easily approximate heel and buttock in the prone position. In general, children should have greater ranges of motion than those indicated on adult range of motion recording forms.

Leg lengths are measured from the anterior superior spine of the pelvis to the medial malleolus of the ipsilateral ankle. An eyeball method which produces reliable results involves positioning the child in supine with hips level. Gentle traction is applied manually to the legs and the length discrepancy between the internal malleoli is measured or judged visually.

Functional Evaluation

Malalignment of joints and movement patterns in both affected and unaffected joints should be observed. Deviations from the norm should be noted and form a basis for the development of a physical therapy program.[26] Pain and bony growth defects can cause the child to assume abnormal postures. Standing posture should be observed from all sides. Leg–length discrepancy may cause a pelvic obliquity and a compensatory scoliosis. An abnormally increased lordosis is common when hip and knee flexion contractures occur, and may persist even when the contractures are reduced. Trunk flexibility should be assessed, particularly in the older child with long-standing disease and in the inactive teenager. Tightness in the low back and hamstrings can combine to cause pain and limit function. When there is prolonged knee inflammation, a valgus deformity frequently develops. The ankles and feet should be checked for proper alignment, including a valgus or varus deformity of the hindfoot and the integrity of the arches. Arthritic involvement of the first metatarsal can produce abnormal flexion in the great toes that only appears in weight bearing.

The child's gait will show an accentuation of the posture noted in standing. Because of the early age of onset in JRA many children never experience normal movement patterns and may continue to use abnormal patterns after disease activity has subsided and normal range of motion of joints is present. In more severe disease this is complicated by bony growth defects which affect posture. At the hip and knee these result in internal rotation of the femur and a valgus deformity at the knee. There may be an accompanying external tibial torsion. Other common gait abnormalities include hip and knee flexion throughout stance and swing phases, decreased movement in hip and/or knee during swing phase, and forward flexion of head and body. A child with a leg–length discrepancy will circumduct the longer leg in swing phase and in stance either hold the leg aligned with the trunk but with hip and knee flexed or externally rotated, abducted, and flexed at the hip, or with hip and knee entended and pelvic obliquity.

Children with severe foot involvement walk on the heel, mid-foot, and lateral metatarsal heads. They do not complete the normal shift on to the medial metatarsal heads and toes, particularly the great toe.[27] Clinically, this results in a shuffling gait.

Positioning of the wrist in extension is very important to maximize hand function. Children with JRA commonly hold the wrist in flexion and avoid placing the hand flat when using the arm for support. Lateral deviation, when seen, is ulnar rather than radial, as in adults with RA. Deviation of the fingers is also reversed with radial deviation being more common in children. Loss of flexion is usual in the MCP joints and loss of extension in the proximal interphalangeal (PIP) and distal interphalangeal (DIP) joints.[28]

When cervical spine involvement is present, the head is frequently held in flexion and the child raises the eyes rather than tipping the head to look at the ceiling. The body rather than the head and neck is turned to look to the side. Mouth opening may be limited where there is temporomandibular joint involvement. The combination of temporomandibular and cervical spine disease may lead to problems with eating and dental hygiene.

A functional assessment for use in JRA has been devised by MacBain and Hill. It includes timed ambulation, grip strength, and putting on and removing socks and a vest.[29]

Physical Therapy Treatment

Modalities

Superficial heating is used in JRA to increase local blood supply and thereby decrease musculoskeletal pain and muscle spasm. The pain threshold may be altered making it easier to perform the exercise program.[30] Heat has been shown to elongate collagen and to give residual elongation when combined with stretching.[31]

For children the most convenient method of applying superficial heat is the home bath tub. The water temperature should be between 98 and 100° F (38° C). Parents are instructed to check the temperature with a fever thermometer. The child should stay in the tub 15 to 20 minutes to experience the desired physiologic response. Both the heat and the bouyancy of the water may assist in the performance of specific exercises in the tub. A whirlpool is not necessary.

Baths are recommended upon arising to help relieve morning stiffness and at bedtime to encourage a more restful night. If the child wakes at night because of aching joints or has increased swelling and tenderness due to a flare, the baths may be given more frequently.

When particular joints are inflamed, direct heat to those joints, either with commercial hot packs or a hot moist towel, well wrung out and covered with plastic and dry towels will provide greater relief of pain than does the tub bath.

Paraffin is an excellent method of providing heat for hands and wrists. However, it is a difficult procedure to carry out at home and great care should be taken in instructing parents and patients in its use. The commercially available paraffin heater is an improvement over double boilers, deep fryers, and crockpots but is expensive. Its use is recommended, however. With very young children who are sensitive to heat, the first few layers may be painted on with a brush. Then the child will usually tolerate dipping the hand to complete the usual 10 or 12 layers.

Superficial cooling by application of cold packs or ice massage is not frequently used in the treatment of JRA. However cold can provide physiologic responses that may be helpful in treating the muscle spasm and pain associated with contracted muscles (i.e., decreased muscle spindle activity and spasm, rebound vasodilatation, and increased pain threshold).[30,31] Swezey states that the more acute the process the more cold will help, and leaves the choice to patient preference.[32] Certainly an acutely swollen, warm joint can be very effectively treated with an ice pack.

Therapeutic Exercise

Active and stretching exercises are necessary parts of an exercise program for children with connective tissue disease. The specifics of exercise programs for juvenile ankylosing spondylitis, dermatomyositis, and scleroderma patients are discussed in the sections on physical therapy in those diseases.

Stretching.   Muscle contractures occur early in JRA because of the self-splinting children do. They place their joints in the position of greatest comfort, usually flexion. If stretching is begun promptly, carried out consistently, and reinforced with the use of resting splints that emphasize extension, the contractures are usually controllable. A common mistake is to discontinue exercise during acute flares. Each affected joint should be taken through at least partial range three to five times each day to maintain range of motion during a flare.

It is recommended that stretching exercises follow a period of tub heat. The child moves the part, with or without assistance, to the point of discomfort. The parent or therapist applies a slight pressure to provide a stretch across the joint. This position is held for a count of 10, then relaxed. The stretching exercises are done twice a day, five to ten times each, depending on the severity of the contracture.

Positioning stretches may also be used, particularly for the hips. A half hour spent lying prone will give an effective stretch to hip and knee flexors if the child is carefully positioned. A wedge cushion under the chest will increase comfort. This position is also used for strengthening of back and neck extensors. Longsitting combined with forward bends gives an effective low back and hamstring stretch. Have the child sit on a cushion if necessary to allow full knee extension and a straight spine.

In patients seen at the University of Michigan Pediatric Rheumatology Clinic this routine has been effective. A general rule used in evaluating the treatment is that pain should not persist more than 2 hours after stretching and the child should not be worse the following day. In actuality pain rarely persists after the treatment periods.

Strengthening. Isometric exercise will maintain muscle strength and bulk and can be safely used during the acute phase of JRA. When the disease is less active, resistance may be used if careful instruction is given in a very gradual program of increasing resistance to avoid joint stress.

Active Exercise. Children's interest in a home program can be heightened and prolonged by imaginative use of activities. It may be necessary to include specific exercises for specific muscles, such as quadriceps, but general conditioning and some specific strengthening can be accomplished by activities.

Swimming provides the best general exercise for children with JRA, because the bouyancy of the water gives support, making movement easier while at the same time giving resistance to movement. It also decreases the stress to the joints that occurs in full weight bearing. Tricycle or bicycle riding also exercises the lower extremities without weight bearing. Propelling a scooter board with the hands gives trunk and wrist extension. Swinging in a prone position provides exercise for various muscle groups depending on the position of arms and legs. Various range of motion dances have been devised and are fun for all ages. Swezey has designed a set of exercises done with a beach ball that appeal to children. It combines range of motion and isometrics.[33]

Activity Regulation. Young children with JRA will usually regulate their activity themselves depending on the state of their disease. Teenagers feeling more peer pressure may need more external structure to help them avoid overtiring and joint stress. Any child with JRA may need increased rest at times but complete bedrest is not advised. It is important to keep these children mobile, participating in school, family, and community life. This provides physiologic and psychologic benefits. If a child quits walking, it is an emergency situation and the rheumatologist should be promptly notified.

Certain activities are discouraged in the interest of joint protection. These include activities that cause the weight of the body to impact on the joints (jumping, hard running); use of pillows that hold a joint in flexion; supporting total body weight on non-weight bearing joints (chin-ups, cartwheels); activities that place stress across a joint (skiing, Indian sitting).

Activities that provide joint protection are encouraged: wearing heels that are 1 inch or less when there is ankle involvement; lifting by using the larger joints; using the palms rather than fingers to grasp heavy objects; using good body mechanics when carrying objects; placing the wrists in neutral or some extension when at rest.[17]

Home Program

In all pediatric rheumatologic conditions a daily exercise program to prevent muscle weakness and/or decreased range of motion is the first priority.[34] Treatment two or three times a week by a physical therapist will not accomplish those goals. Therefore a well designed home program understood and carried out by the child and family is vital.

Swezey has postulated three rules helpful in designing any therapeutic program: (1) the simplest, most efficient, least painful, and least expensive program gets maximum compliance; (2) stretching and strengthening exercises are designed to achieve individual goals that will not be met by general activities; (3) all therapeutic regimens must be monitored.[32]

In any chronic disabling disease of children it is vital to devise a home exercise program that can be carried out by the child and family with the least possible disruption of their daily routine. Occupational and physical therapists should cooperate to design a program that fulfills their combined goals without unnecessary duplication. If the therapists devise a simple method of checking range of motion at home, this can reinforce compliance with the program.

The exercises involved, particularly those that stretch muscles, will cause some discomfort, if not pain, to the child. The parents are often already feeling the guilt that is associated with having a child with chronic illness and may find it very difficult to cause the child more pain. They may also be afraid that the exercises will do damage to the child. Careful structuring and explanation of the home program help insure its being carried out.

Reassure the parents that though almost without exception the 2- or 3-year-old child will cry, that is not a contraindication to treatment. In adults with RA, family expectations have been found to influence compliance with treatment and this is also true with children.[36] If the parents can approach the program as being as much a part of the daily routine as toothbrushing, it will help the child accept it too.

Getting the child involved in the treatment is the first step in gaining cooperation. Moving a bead from one cup to another after each repetition of an exercise helps the 2-year-olds realize that there is a limit to the exercises. Learning to count to 10 can give the child the feeling that he or she controls the length of each stretch. Ritual is comforting to a child and can easily be incorporated in a program.

Even with the youngest children try to include an exercise that they do alone with only supervision from a parent. As the children grow older, restructure the program so they can do the exercises while being supervised by a parent and eventually on their own.

Teenagers present a special problem, especially if their disease is long-standing. In a study of medication compliance in teenagers, those who rated high in self-esteem and autonomy were most compliant. A longer duration of disease and a high number of symptoms present at onset correlated with a poor self-concept and poor compliance.[37] It has been clinically observed that this also applies to carrying out a home exercise program. Certainly an appeal to adult responsibility is in order. Questioning to find out their interests, activities they enjoy, tasks they would like to be able to do for themselves, and activities that their friends are involved in may give clues for designing a program that will appeal to them.

Instruction

Ideally the patient and parents would go through the exercise program several times under the supervision of the therapist. In an outpatient clinic this is not possible so the therapist must give careful instruction, then have the patient and parents actually do the exercises. Oral instruction alone is not enough. If a written program is not given to them at the clinic, have them repeat the exercises before they leave. A written program should be promptly sent. It should make clear which exercises are to stretch and which to strengthen as many people confuse these. The home program should be re-evaluated at each return visit and modified as necessary.

The therapists should also aid in teaching the parents what to expect the child to do as far as activities of daily living are concerned. Maintaining a schedule of activities such as dressing and household chores is important for both functional and psychological outcome. Parents should be aware that the child's ability to participate may vary from day to day according to the degree of disease activity, but encouraging independence will help the child to take a full role in adult society when he or she is grown.

Education

The therapists must be well acquainted with other aspects of the total treatment so that they can answer questions or refer the parent to the proper source. In a well integrated clinic each staff member will ask questions pertaining to other disciplines so that they can reinforce important information and instructions. They also inform the other staff members about areas in specific disciplines in which the family needs more information.

In summary, to encourage participation in and compliance with the home exercise program the therapist should (1) educate the patient and parents regarding the need for and the goals of the program, (2) periodically review the program and change it as needed, (3) provide a means of home evaluation of progress, (4) adapt the program as the child gets older so there is more responsibility in carrying it out, and (5) emphasize the hoped for outcome: that the child will become a responsible, independent adult.

Family, Community and School

If the family is not able to cope with a home program, it may be necessary to make referral for therapy at a local hospital. Often the local therapist may not have had experience with pediatric rheumatologic diseases and may need information on the disease, the treatment, and the expected outcome. Parents and other family members also need to know sources of information. In the case of JRA the only information available at the local library may be on adult arthritis in which the outcome is far less optimistic. At our clinic handbooks are provided covering general information on the disease, the medications the child is most likely to take, the physical and occupational therapy programs, and psychosocial development. The Arthritis Foundation publishes a pamphlet entitled "Arthritis in Childhood."[38] Patients at our clinic are given a pamphlet describing JRA and our clinic's philosophy and methods of treatment.[39]

Most children with JRA are of normal intelligence and should be in a regular classroom at their neighborhood school. It is wise to provide information to school personnel so they can understand the needs of these children. Most will need to take medication during the school day and arrangements may need to be made with the school nurse by the social worker or physician. Therapist consultation with the gym teacher can aid in encouraging the child's participation in as much of the physical education program as is medically approved or in providing an adaptive physical education program. The classroom teacher should be aware that the child with JRA needs to change positions frequently and walk around the room to prevent stiffness. An opportunity for the child to spend some time in the prone position during the school day may contribute to preventing hip and knee flexion contractures. The Arthritis Foundation has a pamphlet specifically written for teachers entitled "When Your Student Has Arthritis."[40]

If therapy is available through the child's school, this can be an important adjunct to the home program. If the school district is one which groups all its services at a central location, this may make it difficult to obtain treatment for the child in the home school but it is important that the child should attend the home school for psychosocial reasons. Therefore the therapy services should accommodate this.

Whitehouse et al[41] surveyed the parents of 152 children with JRA. A total of 135 of the children were attending school, of these one quarter had problems with mobility, fine motor hand skills, and upper extremity activities in school. The most common difficulty was writing and the next was getting to class on time. A second study found that a visit to the school by a health professional specifically involved in the child's care was the preferred way of gaining information. Communication with an informed parent was second and resource materials third.[42]

Orthoses

Orthoses are prescribed by a physician but the occupational and physical therapists are involved in the decision and are most likely to check on continued use, fit, and effectiveness. The orthoses used in connective tissue disease are of three types: resting, functional and corrective.[43]

Resting Orthoses. The purpose of the resting or positioning orthosis is to provide the beneficial effects of rest and support for inflamed joints. Because children ankylose more readily than adults, emphasis is placed on positioning for maximum function. The joint is placed in as much extension as the patient's range of motion permits. One of the most commonly used resting orthoses is the wrist-hand orthosis. It is prescribed when there is continued inflammation with loss of range. It is made of heat-moldable plastic and is usually fitted directly on the child rather than by taking a cast and vacuum molding. If finger joints are involved, support can be extended just past the metacarpophalangeal (MCP) joints or to the end of the fingers. Flexion contractures of the PIP and DIP joints respond well to the stretch provided by having the child wear an orthosis with a resting pan for the fingers. The orthosis can be padded to provide varying degrees of extension for each finger joint.

If only one finger joint is involved, or if there is a swan neck or boutonniére type of deformity, a ring splint may help in gaining normal range and function or preventing further deformity.

Early use of a resting orthosis on knees and elbows may help prevent the development of flexion contractures. They are made similarly to the wrist-hand orthosis with the joint placed in as much extension as is comfortable for the child.

To prevent interference with normal activity, resting orthoses are worn at night. This also keeps the child from assuming a flexed position during sleep. Though the splints are not designed to provide a stretch, range of motion is sometimes increased with consistent use. If a joint is in flare, the orthosis may be worn during the day for increased support and comfort.

Cervical collars are used in JRA when there is cervical spine involvement. If there is no radiologic evidence of subluxation, a soft collar is used. It provides support, aids in reducing associated muscle spasm, and may help prevent a fixed flexion deformity.[17] If there is subluxation, a more rigid collar is prescribed. It is worn during the day and a soft collar worn at night. Bony fusion frequently occurs and a functional head position is maintained by using the collar. It is especially important to protect the cervical spine during active play and while riding in a motor vehicle. Neither the soft nor the rigid collar provide immobilization of the cervical spine.[44] They do position the head in a neutral position, relieve pain, and remind the child not to stress the cervical spine.

Functional Orthoses. Functional orthoses are used to support a joint during activity. Sometimes a resting orthosis can also be used as a functional orthosis as is the case with cervical collars. In our clinic we rarely order functional orthoses for the wrist or knee. This is partly an economic issue. We regularly use resting orthoses and third–party payers are reluctant to cover two splints for the same joint. Also we want the child to be as active and using muscles as freely as possible during the day. If a child is having discomfort during daily activities, we may suggest using the resting splint if it allows functional movement. When there is severe ulnar deviation of the wrist, a wrist-hand orthosis with a joint that allows flexion and extension but not ulnar deviation may be used during the day.

Lifts and other shoe adaptations are used commonly and are necessary in many cases to improve function. When knee and/or ankle joints are involved, careful watch must be kept for a leg–length discrepancy. If one develops that is 1.5 cm or more, a lift is ordered that will be equal to one half of the leg length difference. This lift may be inside the heel of the shoe or on the sole. If the lift must be higher than 0.5 cm, it cannot be accommodated entirely inside the shoe. For an appearance conscious teenager, a more cosmetic effect can be gained by using a heel lift in one shoe and cutting down the heel on the other shoe. A lift may be used even though hips are level and spine straight if there is even a small flexion contracture of the knee. With a one eighth or one quarter inch lift, full extension may be achieved.

Scaphoid and metatarsal pads are used to provide support and relieve pressure on involved joints. The metatarsal pads are placed proximally to the heads of the metarsals so that weight is born on the shaft of the bone rather than on the joints. If the pads are not enough to relieve pain in these joints, a metatarsal bar may be added to the bottom of the shoe. If the child is toeing in or out in ambulation because of pain in the foot, a Thomas or reverse Thomas heel may correct this. If more correction is needed, a sole wedge may be added. Two or three tongue blades taped to the sole of the shoe provide an easy way to evaluate if a wedge will be effective.

A molded plastic ankle-foot orthosis may be indicated if there are multiple problems in alignment and gait disturbances. Scaphoid and metatarsal pads can be incorporated in the orthosis. If it is the foot that needs support, a flat–bottomed insert that comes high enough to firmly support the heel may be enough. If the ankle is also a problem, the orthosis should be brought up to just below the knee. These orthoses have the added advantage that they can be worn in a variety of shoes. Extra depth shoes are not available in most childrens' sizes, which often makes placing pads in shoes difficult. However, in the child who is growing quickly the cost of frequent replacements of an orthosis may be prohibitive.

As to shoes, a proper fit in a comfortable yet supportive shoe is the basic requirement. If orthotic work needs to be done on the shoe, a leather shoe may be required. For many children a well-cushioned sports shoe that can be fastened securely and has a built-in arch support is both comfortable and therapeutic.

Corrective Orthoses. An orthosis designed to increase movement at a joint may use either a turnbuckle or elastics. Turnbuckles work well until the flexion contracture is reduced to 20° or less. Then they are at a mechanical disadvantage. They are heavy and uncomfortable and can usually only be used for two or three half–hour periods during the day, though occasionally a child will sleep in one. A dynamic extension splint uses elastics to pull the joint into extension. The amount of tension can be adjusted so that the child can flex the joint but there is a constant pull to extension. The dynamic splints are usually lightweight and well tolerated. As a general rule the turnbuckles will be used to help stretch out stubborn flexion contractures and a dynamic splint used to continue and maintain the progress. The extra support of knee extension given by the dynamic splint encourages ambulation in some children.

Dynamic hand splints are not often used in our clinic. Young children do not tolerate them but in an older child when there is severe limitation of flexion at the MCP joints, a knuckle-bender type of orthosis may be indicated.

Adaptive Equipment

A wide range of adaptive equipment may be used to make the severely involved child as independent as possible. Activities of daily living aids such as long-handled bath sponges or hair brushes, dressing sticks, or reachers help in achieving independence. Crutches or canes may be needed to relieve lower extremity joints. If there is also upper extremity involvement, forearm platforms rather than hand grips should be used. Great care must be taken not to increase upper extremity problems in trying to relieve those in the lower extremities.

Wheelchair use is avoided as long as possible because of the importance of continuing ambulation to maintain muscle and bony strength. A collapsible buggy is lightweight, easily handled, and a help on long outings. However, as children approach the teenage years, a wheelchair may be seen by them as more socially acceptable. The very lightweight chairs made by the sports chair companies are preferred for their adaptability and ease of maneuverability. There is a strong case to be made for allowing a severely involved child the independence of movement gained by using a manual wheelchair or electric vehicle. However, a careful assessment of the child and family should be made by the rheumatology team before suggesting such a move in order to avoid the situation in which the vehicle is accepted as the only means of movement for the child.

Orthopedic Surgery

The orthopedic surgeon may be called on to help in the management of patients where the usual treatment of anti-inflammatory medicine and physical therapy has not prevented joint deformity. Various modes of orthopedic treatment may be used. In general, operative procedures are delayed to allow for full bone growth, better patient cooperation, and perhaps remission of the inflammatory disease.[7]

Serial Casting

Serial casting is most commonly used for knee flexion contractures. The regimen usually consists of cast changes every 2 to 4 days with slight correction of the deformity at each change.[45,46] Care must be taken to avoid forced extension of the joint.[6] When full extension is reached or there is no more progress, the cast may be bivalved so that physical therapy may be done out of the cast.

Traction

Traction may be used when both knees and hips are contracted or for knees alone. Skin traction can be an important adjunct to a vigorous physical and occupational therapy program in the hospital. In some severe knee flexion contractures balanced skeletal traction will gain extension.[46]

Synovectomy

Synovectomy is not often used in JRA. There is a high possibility of spontaneous remission. If there is a flare instead of remission, there is likelihood that synovitis will reoccur. The most consistent good result is the relief of pain.[47] Range of motion increased in less than half of the joints operated on in two studies.[47,48] The greatest success of synovectomy reported in one study was in large joints that were boggy and swollen.[49] This group stated that synovectomy is "very rarely indicated . . . but does have an appropriate place in the treatment of children." At the University of Michigan synovectomy has not been used for the past 12 years.

Joint Fusion

Ankylosis of joints occurs due to the disease process, particularly in the wrists and cervical spine. If these joints have been held in proper positions by physical therapy and splinting, function will be maintained. In the older teenager surgical fusion of a subluxed wrist or thumb MCP joint may provide a functional grasp. Surgical fusion of the cervical spine is done only for progressive neurologic signs.[50] If a joint has fused in a non-functional position or if there is malalignment of bones because of growth defects, osteotomy may be indicated.

Soft Tissue Release

Soft tissue release may be needed to gain range of motion and functional position in contracted joints that have not responded to medication and physical therapy. This is particularly true when iliotibial band tightness is contributing to knee flexion and genu valgum. Releases may be done either before or during joint replacement procedures to gain range of motion.[51]

Joint Replacement Surgery

Joint replacement surgery is becoming more common in adolescent and young adult patients who have had deforming JRA over a number of years. The small size of many of the joints means that special joint components are required. If there is severe osteoporosis or if upper extremity function is poor, hip and knee replacement may not be advised.[52,53] The child must have been functional enough to have maintained muscle strength. The grade of strength required has not been specifically documented. The life expectancy of the joint components becomes particularly important when they are placed in a younger patient. Twenty to 30 years is the current estimate. It is felt that because the patients with JRA who are considered for joint replacement are smaller and less active than the adult patients, they may place less stress on the components resulting in longer wear.[45,53,54]

Relief of pain is less often the reason for joint replacement in JRA than it is in adult arthritis.[45,53] Indications for replacement surgery in JRA are a significant functional limitation, and the presence of a fixed deformity. Where there has been pain, it is generally relieved postoperatively and some increase of functional status is gained.[45,55] If multiple joint replacements are needed, the patient's functional status wil generally improve but will not approach normal.[55] Extensive pre- and postoperative physical therapy is needed to obtain the best outcome.

When both hips and knees have fixed deformities, most surgeons prefer to operate on the hips first. Because of the growth defects of JRA in the femur, an osteotomy is often needed. Soft tissue releases around the hip are usually done too. These do not add significantly to the range of motion, but when combined with a physical therapy program, range of motion, strength, and ability to ambulate are improved.[45,55] The main component problem postoperatively is loosening. This happens in the acetabular component in JRA as opposed to the femoral component in adults.[56]

After the hips have been treated, some knees can be improved with serial casting. If there is a severe fixed deformity (>45°) the knees may be replaced first. A careful assessment of bone size is necessary to determine if joint components can be successfully placed. Extensive posterior soft tissue release is usually required. A combined deformity of valgus and flexion which frequently occurs in JRA is very difficult to correct.[51]

The surgeon's job is made easier if the patient has continued to be as active as possible over the years. Even limited ambultion can help maintain muscle strength and bone density. Many children with severe JRA (and their parents) look forward to joint replacement as a magic operation that will solve many problems. They should be made aware of the limited improvement possible and of the year or so of hard work in physical therapy needed to make maximal gains. Before surgery is done, careful counseling and evaluation with the patient and family is needed to assess their understanding of the procedures and probable outcome, their motivation for wanting surgery, and their ability to cooperate in the total program.[53,54]

Surgical procedures are done in an attempt to bring the child toward a more normal functional status. Unlike adults with rheumatoid arthritis, the child with severe JRA has probably never experienced normality and must make many adjustments, both physical and psychological, if there is to be maximum benefit from surgery.[52]

Physical Therapy

The first requisite is that a physical therapist shall have been involved with the patient over the years redesigning the home program as needed and encouraging the child and family to continue working to maintain range of motion and strength. Helping the family find ways for the child or young adult to continue at least partial ambulating and to spend some portion of the day in the prone position may prevent or delay the time when use of a wheelchair for mobility becomes necessary. If a young person is using a wheelchair or electric vehicle, it is very important to help the family arrange the school program so that some time may be spent standing or prone during the school day.

When it becomes clear that joint replacement or other orthopedic surgery will be performed, the physical therapist should help in the counseling of the patient by explaining what the sequence of exercise and ambulation will be. Patients and their families should be made to realize that to gain maximum benefits from the surgery the physical therapy program may need to be continued up to one year.

Immediately preoperatively the patient and family should be instructed in the exercises designed for the early postoperative period. This should help in gaining cooperation at a time when the child is experiencing pain and discomfort from the surgery. If there is arthritis in joints other than the operated ones, exercise for these joints should be part of the daily program while in the hospital.

The specific progression of weight bearing, ambulation, and exercise desired may vary from one institution to another. Ansell[57] describes some general principles which can be seen in knee and hip surgeries. After knee surgery, extension is maintained by the cast. Flexion may be slow to be regained. After a supracondylar osteotomy, the children are casted for an extended period of time. Again flexion will be regained slowly. She suggests that children who have had knee surgery use a tricycle or bicycle for transport, not a wheelchair.

For soft tissue releases, hydrotherapy after cast removal will aid in regaining mobility. Hydrotherapy is also used after total hip replacements after the wound has healed. These patients have weak hip and back muscles because ambulation may have been limited for many years. They may need a period of treatment with strengthening exercise and progressive ambulation training before they are ready to use crutches. They should continue to use crutches until they can walk without a Trendelenberg limp. She suggests that they continue to receive weekly physical therapy as range of motion and strength improve. This may take up to 1 year. After maximum improvement is achieved, it should be maintained by a regular program of exercise designed by the physical therapist.

It is not enough to merely teach an exercise program. The patient should also be taught how to use the improved function in daily life. For the severely involved child some activities may now be possible that had not been experienced before. These suggestions also apply to recovery after fractures of the lower extremity.

JUVENILE ANKYLOSING SPONDYLITIS

Symptoms and Diagnosis

Although thought of as a disease of young adult males, ankylosing spondylitis can occur in childhood. Increasing reports of this disease entity are appearing in the literature, and it seems likely that more childhood cases will be recognized.

The typical early symptoms include pain in the low back, hips, buttocks, or thighs. This pain may be mild and intermittent, appearing first on one side and then the other. Enthesitis, or pain at the insertion of tendons and ligaments to bones, is very common and an indicator that a diagnosis of juvenile ankylosing spondylitis (JAS) should be considered.[58] Frequently there may be associated arthritis of one or more peripheral joints. This arthritis is usually nondeforming, most frequently affecting knees and ankles. These bouts of pain and stiffness may come and go for several years. Indeed, patients who have been diagnosed in their early 20s have been able retrospectively to trace symptoms to onset in childhood.[59]

Diagnosis depends on (1) symptoms of sacroiliac joint or low back pain, (2) demonstrable decreased mobility of the lumbar or lumbodorsal spine, and (3) radiographic sacroiliac changes.[59] There is no definitive laboratory test and, in contrast to adults, most children do not have spine or sacroiliac symptoms at onset.[58] Because of this it is often not possible to diagnose JAS for several years. If there is peripheral joint involvement, a diagnosis of JRA is commonly made first.

Sex incidence is reported variably but is approximately six males to one female in contrast to the other pediatric rheumatologic diseases where the incidence ratio is reversed.[58] An acute iritis (in contrast to the chronic uveitis of JRA) frequently occurs and may aid in diagnosis. Amyloidosis is seen frequently in adults with ankylosing spondylitis (AS) but rarely in children in North America. Cardiac disease occurs in 5 percent of adults followed 15 years after onset. It is much rarer in children but this may reflect the shorter length of follow-up.[58]

Spondylitis, similar to JAS, can be associated with other diseases including inflammatory bowel disease, Reiter's disease, and psoariasis.

Genetic Factors

No cause is known, but a definite genetic linkage was found with the identification in 1974 of a specific gene, HLA-B27. This is present in 90 percent of patients with ankylosing spondylitis, as opposed to 7 to 8 percent of the general population. It is present in 50 percent of the first-degree relatives of these patients.[60]

Histocompatibility antigens are present on the surface of most body cells. The differences in these antigens from one individual to another are responsible for tissue rejections in organ graft procedures. Human leukocyte antigens (HLA) are one type of histocompatibility antigen. They react with antigens on the surface of human leukocytes to cause agglutination. The particular gene associated with ankylosing spondylitis in the HLA chromosome system is B27. That is, it is one of the 26 different genes which may occur at the B–locus on human chromosome number six.

Individuals who carry the histocompatibility antigen HLA-B27 are 30 to 200 times more at risk for arthritis of the sacroiliac joints or spine than the general population.[60] However, probably fewer than 10 percent of those who carry HLA-B27 will ever have symptoms of ankylosing spondylitis.[59] Therefore its presence is helpful in making a definite diagnosis but cannot be considered as diagnostic by itself.

Radiologic Joint Changes

Radiographically the normal sacroiliac joints of childhood and adolescence are wider than the adult joints with naturally serrated margins which are lacking in articular cortex. Between 17 and 20 years of age they gradually change to the narrower, smoother adult type of joint. The articular cortex appears as a white line on radiographs of mature joints.

In adult ankylosing spondylitis the sacroiliac joints appear similar to the healthy adolescent joint. In adolescents the involved joints show large subcortical erosions which give the appearance of widening of the joint space. Periarticular sclerosis results in increased density along the sides of the joint. This sclerosis may be the first radiologic sign to appear and is sometimes overlooked. Involvement of the spine cannot be positively diagnosed until squaring of the vertebral bodies is evident.[61] This change is rare in children and adolescents but will occur in adults after childhood onset.[58]

Etiology

The discovery of the genetically determined character of JAS has stimulated several speculations but precise etiology is unknown. It may be triggered by infection or the failure of normal response to infection. JAS is similar to other spondyloarthropathies that are triggered by bacterial infection suggesting a similar mechanism although none has been found.[58]

Medical Treatment

The goals of treatment of JAS are similar to those of JRA, namely, to provide control of pain and inflammation, to prevent deformity, and to educate the patient, family, and community in order to insure as functional an outcome as possible.[62,63] If a prior diagnosis of JRA has been made, a careful discussion of the diagnostic process, the likelihood that the disease will continue into adulthood, and the need for long-term medications, physical therapy, and follow-up is needed to assure understanding and compliance with treatment. It is well to stress that careful medication and a conscientiously practised exercise program can lead to a good functional prognosis.[58]

Drug Therapy

Aspirin is sufficient to control pain and reduce inflammation in some cases and should be tried before other medications. If the patient does not respond to salicylates, indomethacin may offer a good response.

Prognosis

Prognosis depends on whether the disease progresses to involve most of the spine or arrests early. If an erect posture is maintained, good functional ability is possible even with fusion of the entire spine. About 75 percent of patients in one series of 311 adults with ankylosing spondylitis were in functional Classes I and II. Only five were confined to bed or chair.[62] The peripheral arthritis that occurs with childhood onset may cause more disability, especially if the hips are involved.[63] The acute iritis usually responds well to treatment.

The chance of a JAS patient with HLA-B27 having a male child with JAS is approximately 5 percent and even less for a female child.[58]

Physical Therapy

Evaluation

The peripheral joints involved in JAS are commonly diagnosed first as JRA and are treated in that manner. Hamstring, hip flexor, and low back tightness are common. Mobility of the spine must be assessed. Forward bending is best measured using Schober's test.[64] Frost et al, found forward and side bending and prone knee flexion were accurately measured in centimeters.[65] Back bending, trunk rotation, and straight leg raising were not reliably measured by their technique. A second person to help in positioning for straight leg raising, and the lighter weight of children's legs might make that measurement more accurate.

Measurement of chest expansion should be carried out early to aid in detection of involvement of costovertebral joints. In the adolescent less than 5 cm excursion is suspect.[58] Serial measurements should be made to follow progress.

Posture should be observed on a regular basis. The maintenance of an erect posture with as normal an alignment as possible is critical in insuring a good functional outcome for the patient. The contour of the back in forward bending should be observed for flattening of the lumbosacral spine.[58]

Treatment

The primary goal of physical therapy is to maintain flexibility and an erect posture.[62] Emphasis is placed on maintaining range of motion in hips, shoulders, and spine. Lateral and forward flexion of the spine should be included as well as extension. Deep breathing for chest expansion is taught. If the chest cavity becomes fixed, instruction in abdominal breathing may be an important aid in respiration. Strengthening of spine and hip extensors aids in maintaining the erect posture.

Painful enthesitis at the insertion of the Achilles tendon and the plantar fascia may be relieved by the use of molded insoles which take pressure off the plantar surface of the heel and the metarsal heads.[58] The elimination of a pillow and use of a bedboard are desirable.[62]

Patients with JAS with accompanying hip disease may have a poorer functional prognosis than those who have only spinal involvement.[63] This emphasizes the need for particular attention to exercises for maintaining hip mobility. Hip arthroplasty has not been as successful in patients with JAS as in those with JRA.[66] Pain must be relieved by the proper anti-inflammatory agent before compliance with an exercise program can be expected.[62]

DERMATOMYOSITIS

Dermatomyositis of childhood is an uncommon inflammatory disease of unknown etiology, which affects striated muscle, skin, and blood vessels. More rarely the gastrointestinal tract and other internal organs may be involved. It is not associated with malignancy in children as it is in adults. The ratio of females to males is 2:1. It is seen more often in children than is polymyositis.[67] Pearson distinguished it as a separate category in his 1966 classification of dermatomyositis and polymyositis.[68]

Onset can occur any time during childhood, but is most frequent during the first decade. Onset can be acute, subacute, or chronic. Usually there is gradual weakening of the proximal muscles evidenced by increased falling or difficulty climbing stairs. There may be muscle pain and tenderness and, less frequently, arthralgias. Fever and general malaise, combined with the parents' recognition of the child's loss of function due to weakness, lead to seeking medical advice. Some children have periorbital edema. Approximately 10 percent of the children develop dysphagia and dyspnea. Careful watch should be kept for these symptoms so that respiratory assistance can be provided if needed.[67,69,70]

The skin involvement is evidenced by a distinctive rash which is seen in 75 percent of the patients. There is a heliotrope (purplish) or erythematous discoloration of eyelids, cheeks, and extensor surfaces of joints, particularly MCP and PIP joints. The underlying lesion is a vasculitis. The progression of the rash to a diffuse, generalized vasculitis is a poor prognostic sign.[67]

Calcinosis, or subcutaneous deposits of calcium salts, is usually a late symptom which occurs in 40 percent of patients.[67] Disability depends on the size and location of the deposits. Small nodules may break through the skin and drain. Larger areas may require surgical excision if they hinder joint mobility or are over pressure areas. In a small number of severe cases *calcinosis universalis* may occur in which the body develops an exoskeleton of calcium deposits.

Diagnosis

Clinical diagnosis is made in the presence of proximal muscle weakness and pain and the pathognomic rash. It is confirmed by abnormally increased serum levels of muscle enzymes, muscle biopsy showing signs of inflammatory myositis, and electromyography demonstrating myopathic units, fibrillation, and denervation potential.[67]

Recent research suggests a disturbance of the immune system may be responsible for some of the symptoms of this disease, but as yet, etiology is unknown.

Medical Treatment

When the diagnosis is made, the child is started on a course of high dose corticosteroids. Prednisone is the drug of choice because other steroids have myopathic side effects. The risks of long term steroid use are well known, and to avoid them a taper of the medicine is begun as soon as medically possible. Enzyme levels usually return to normal within 2 weeks after steroids are begun. When they have remained normal for 3 months, a gradual taper is begun. Treatment will be continued for 2 years but at reduced dosages where side effects are less.[67,70,71] Approximately 20 percent of the children will have an exacerbation if the taper is too rapid or if other infection intervenes. Fewer than 10 percent of the children will be unresponsive to steroid therapy or develop steroid toxicity. Other forms of immunosuppressive therapy have been tried with some success in these children. Their use is considered experimental and informed consent must be obtained before they are tried.

Prognosis

In the 1950s one third of patients recovered, one third were disabled due to weakness and muscle contractures, and one third died.[72] With vigorous corticosteroid treatment, mortality has declined to less than 10 percent.[67,73]

Eighty percent of the children treated in the University of Michigan clinic have had a single episode of the disease and recover with normal or near normal function. The other 20 percent have a more chronic course. One half of these resemble polyvasculitis with widespread cutaneous involvement. A minority of patients have involvement of the gastrointestinal tract.[67]

Physical Therapy Treatment

Evaluation

Baseline measurements of muscle strength and range of motion are made at the first patient visit and consistently re-evaluated at subsequent visits. Usually serum enzyme levels begin to fall within 2 weeks after steroid therapy is begun and strength begins to return in 2 to 8 weeks.[67] The child and the parents become aware of an increase in endurance and functional ability. Too frequent formal muscle tests at this point may be discouraging because test grades will not rise rapidly. However, an informal evaluation of strength such as getting down to the floor and up, stepping up a step, and raising arms (with or without resistance) should be done at each visit. If all is going well, a formal muscle test every third month will show progression in strength. If there is an exacerbation of dermatomyositis or any other medical problem, more frequent muscle tests should be done. If available, evaluation using Cybex (Lumex Inc., Ronkonkoma, NY) gives an objective record of muscle strength.

Exercise

Depending on the severity of onset the child may be allowed to continue usual activities with increased rest periods or may be placed on bed rest. In any event, until muscle enzymes return to normal, only passive exercises are used to maintain range of motion. At this stage the child may be depressed and unwilling to cooperate with a physical therapy program.[74] When enzymes are stabilized at a normal level, the child can begin a more active program aimed at regaining functional independence at an age-appropriate level.[67]

Contractures may develop during the acute phase of the disease. They should decrease with gentle stretching, but resting splints should be used early if there is suspicion that the course of the disease may be severe. The child, parents, and nursing staff should be instructed in positioning to increase extension and prevent flexion contractures.

Stretching should be avoided in areas of calcium deposits because of the risk of skin breakdown. Very few children develop the most severe form of dermatoyositis, but in these cases contractures may develop in spite of a conscientious physical therapy program.[75]

Hydrotherapy

If it does not cause an exacerbation of the rash, hydrotherapy may be used in the early stages of the disease to decrease muscle pain and tenderness. If the child is very weak, the tub may allow more movement when active exercise is begun. Where there are extensive subcutaneous deposits of calcium, the skin over these areas may become eroded. There is poor healing because of the inflammatory involvement of skin and blood vessels, and hydrotherapy may be used in this instance to clean and debride these wounds.

Home Program

The program will include stretching of joints where range of motion is limited by muscle contractures and strengthening exercises. At first, it may be enough to allow the child to gain strength by gradually increasing the activity level. A once a week swimming or dancing class can be fun and therapeutic. This works best with younger children. If specific muscles are slow to gain strength, a program should be written that emphasizes them. For older children and teenagers, it is probably best to give them a written program of exercise to strengthen trunk and proximal limb muscles as soon as they are medically ready for it.

Children who have a chronic course of dermatomyositis are particularly at risk for the development of contractures and permanent loss of strength. They will need to have their exercise program consistently re-evaluated in light of the changing status of their disease.

SCLERODERMA

Scleroderma is a disease of connective tissue characterized by vascular, fibrotic, and inflammatory changes in the skin and internal organs. It has been classified into systemic and linear forms with a good prognosis associated with the linear form. However, a linear onset does not preclude development of systemic symptoms. Scleroderma occurs more often in females than in males. The disease in children follows a course similar to that seen in adults.[77]

Systemic Sclerosis

The most common complaint at presentation is tightening of the skin. There may first be edema of the fingers and toes, though this is rare in children. The skin then becomes indurated with loss of pliability, thickening, and tightness. It appears shiny and smooth. A generalized hyperpigmentation with areas of localized depigmentation may be present. Tightening of the skin of the face gives a typical facies including a pinched nose, thin lips, small mouth, and prominent incisors.[77,78] Raynaud's phenomenon is frequent and can occur long before other symptoms. Ulcers frequently form over bony prominences. Resorption of the bony tufts of the digits may occur.[79,80]

In one review of 15 patients the most commonly seen symptoms of organ involvement were Raynaud's phenomenon, contractures, abnormal esophageal mobility, and abnormal pulmonary diffusion. Organ systems involved include skin, digital arteries, musculoskeletal, gastrointestinal tract, lungs, and heart.[80]

There must be visceral involvement for the diagnosis of systemic sclerosis to be made.[81] The course of the disease is very slowly progressive. Diagnostic procedures such as pulmonary diffusion studies, plethysmograpy, and radiographic studies may show that internal organs are affected before clinical symptoms are evident. Earlier diagnosis of systemic involvement may be possible if such studies are done in both the systemic and linear types of onset.[78]

Localized Scleroderma

A lump in the skin is usually the first symptom of localized scleroderma. The area may be edematous and either erythematous or bluish. It gradually becomes sclerotic. If it remains small and circumscribed, it is termed morphea. The usual linear pattern is to spread along one limb, but it can be more generalized. Both types of lesions are seen in one patient.

Widespread linear lesions have a more severe effect on underlying tissue and may be associated with more abnormal laboratory studies.[79] The combination of atrophy and scarring of involved areas next to areas of normal childhood growth produce more contractures and deformities in children than in adults.[82] There may be involvement of the internal organs in addition to the cutaneous manifestations.

Prognosis

Prognosis depends on the systems involved. Some children have improved spontaneously but most have a slowly progressive course. A complete remission has not been reported.[77,79]

Medical Treatment

Dabich prefers the term "patient management" because there is no known agent to cure scleroderma.[77] Treatment depends on the system involved. It is important to allow patients and their families opportunity to vent their feelings about the limitations of activity and the physical disfigurement caused by the disease. Raynaud's phenomenon may be alleviated by vasodilators or, as is common practice today, by drugs that effect sympathetic blockade.

There is a high incidence of decreased esophageal mobility. These children should be on a program to minimize the chance of gastrointestinal reflux by (1) raising the head of the bed 8 inches; (2) not lying down for at least 20 minutes after eating; (3) chewing carefully and using fluids to help increase the ease of swallowing; (4) eating more frequent, smaller meals; (5) using antacids; and (6) learning relaxation techniques to help become calm before meals.[77,83]

Plastic surgery has been used in adults to increase range of motion and function.[84] Operative sites can contract again and need further surgeries in adults. This is even more likely in growing children. Skin grafting to accelerate healing of ulceration and amputation to remove irremediably damaged parts are the surgical role in treatment of the sclerodermatous hand.[85] In children amputation may be the treatment of choice of a severely involved limb.

Physical Therapy

Evaluation

Linear measurement of localized lesions may be used to follow their progression. Location and extent of ulcerated areas should be recorded. Linear involvement of the lower extremities may cause a leg–length discrepancy which should be monitored by careful measurement. Goniometric measurements are done if joint movement is affected. Evaluation of the functional use of the hands and limbs becomes important if there is atrophy, contracture, or painful ulcers present. Muscle testing will aid in determining the effectiveness of prescribed exercises in combating the weakness that may accompany atrophy. Gait and habitual posture should be observed. Melvin et al.[35] suggest that heat may not help all patients to gain range. Pre- and post-heat measurements will aid in determining if heat should be included as a part of the home program.

Treatment

Heat. Warm soaks are used to increase the circulation in the involved areas. They can serve to promote healing of ulcerated areas, and as heat before stretching exercises. Following immersion a lanolin cream should be applied to the sclerotic skin to prevent excessive drying. Because of the vascular involvement, great care must be taken to avoid burning these patients. The temperatures required to melt paraffin may be tolerated only early in the disease. Conversely, because of the high incidence of Raynaud's phenomenon, use of cold is contraindicated.[77]

Exercise. Stretching exercises must be done faithfully several times a day to allow improvement but good results are possible.[86] Providing the patient with an objective method of home evaluation of range of motion allows daily checks and a shifting emphasis in the home program to regain small losses.[35]

In the long term, contractures may develop in spite of a consistent exercise program.

Strengthening exercises are also an important part of a home program because of the severe atrophy that eventually occurs. In order to maintain muscle tone, active resistive exercise should be started early and continued as long as there is progression of the disease.[79,85] In systemic sclerosis the muscles of the face should be exercised to maintain mobility and adequate mouth opening and to delay progression of the typical tight expressionless facies.[35]

Orthoses and Adaptive Equipment. Splints to maintain range of motion gained by surgery or stretching exercises may be needed. They may be worn at night or for specific intervals during the day. Protective pads over calcium deposits or ulcers on bony prominences may be needed for pressure relief. If hand use is limited by ulcers, increased sensitivity, or contractures, dressing or other functional aids can help promote independence.

REFERENCES

1. Petty RE: Epidemiology and genetics of rheumatic diseases of childhood. p. 15. In Cassidy JT (ed): Textbook of Pediatric Rheumatology. John Wiley & Sons, New York, 1982
2. Diagnostic and Therapeutic Criteria Committee, American Rheumatism Association: Criteria for the classification of juvenile rheumatoid arthritis. Bull Rheum Dis 23:712, 1973
3. Ragsdale CG, Petty RE, Cassidy JT, Sullivan DB: The clinical progression of apparent juvenile rheumatoid arthritis to systemic lupus erythematosis. J Rheumatol 7:50, 1980
4. Sullivan DB, Cassidy JT, Petty RE: Pathogenic implications of age of onset in juvenile rheumatoid arthritis. Arthritis Rheum 18:251, 1975
5. Cassidy JT: Juvenile rheumatoid arthritis. p. 1247. In Kelley WN, Harris, ED, Ruddy S, Sledge CB (eds): Textbook of Rheumatology. Vol. II. WB Saunders Co, Philadelphia, 1981
6. Cassidy JT: Juvenile rheumatoid arthritis. In Cassidy, JT (ed): Textbook of Pediatric Rheumatology. John Wiley & Sons, New York, 1982
7. Calabro JJ: Management of juvenile rheumatoid arthritis. J Pediatr 77:355, 1970
8. Bernstein BH, Stobie D, Singsen BH, et al: Growth retardation in juvenile rheumatoid arthritis. Arthritis Rheum (suppl) 20:212, 1977
9. Chylak LT Jr: The ocular manifestations of juvenile rheumatoid arthritis. Arthritis Rheum (suppl) 20:217, 1977
10. Maldonado-Cocco JA, Garcia O, Spindler AJ et al: Carpal ankylosis in juvenile rheumatoid arthritis. Arthritis Rheum 11:1251, 1980
11. Cassidy JT, Martel W: Juvenile rheumatoid arthritis: Clinicoradiologic correlations. Arthritis Rheum (suppl) 20:207, 1977
12. Isdale IC: Hip disease in juvenile rheumatoid arthritis. Ann Rheum Dis 29:603, 1970
13. Cassidy JT, Brady GL, Martel W: Monoarticular juvenile rheumatoid arthritis. J Pediatr 70:867, 1967
14. Ansell B, Wood, PHN: Prognosis in juvenile chronic polyarthritis. Clin Rheum Dis 2:397, 1976

15. Miller JJ, Spitz P, Simpson U, Williams GF: The social function of young adults who had arthritis in childhood. J Pediatr 100:378, 1981
16. Schaller JG, Wedgwood RJ: Juvenile rheumatoid arthritis: A review. Pediatrics 50:940, 1972
17. Sullivan DB: The pediatric rheumatology clinic. p. 615. In Cassidy JT: Textbook of Pediatric Rheumatology. John Wiley & Sons, New York, 1982
18. Stillman JS: Salicylates—a review. Arthritis Rheum (suppl) 20:510, 1977
19. Brewer EJ Jr: Drug therapy. p. 180. In Brewer EJ Jr (ed): Juvenile Rheumatoid Arthritis. WB Saunders, Philadelphia, 1970
20. Levinson JE, Bolz GP, Bondi S: Gold therapy. Arthritis Rheum 20:531, 1977
21. Boone JE, Baldwin J, and Levine C: Juvenile rheumatoid arthritis. Pediatr Clin North Am 21:855, 1974
22. Schaller JG: Corticosteroids in juvenile rheumatoid arthritis. Arthritis Rheum (suppl) 20:537, 1977
23. Sinclair RJG: Corticosteroid therapy in rheumatoid arthritis and other connective tissue disorders. p. 229. In Dixon AS (ed): Progress in Clinical Rheumatology. Little, Brown, Boston, 1965
24. Scott PJ, Ansell BM, Huskisson EC: Measurement of pain in juvenile chronic arthritis. Ann Rheum Dis 36:186, 1977
25. Beales JG, Keen JH, Holt, PJL: The child's perception of the disease and the experience of pain in juvenile chronic arthritis. J Rheumatol 10:61, 1983
26. Barkley E, Brewer EJ Jr: Home treatment program. p. 132. In Brewer EJ Jr (ed): Juvenile Rheumatoid Arthritis. WB Saunders, Philadelphia, 1970
27. Dhanendran M, Hutton WC, Klenerman L, et al: Foot function in juvenile chronic arthritis. Rheumatol Tindall 19:20, 1980
28. Baldwin J: Movement in the hands of children with arthritis. Physiotherapy 61:208, 1975
29. MacBain KP, Hill RH: A functional assessment for juvenile rheumatoid arthritis. Am J Occup Ther 26:326, 1973
30. Figley BA, Danek CJ: Physical therapy in arthritis. Division of Rheumatology, University of Michigan Hospitals, 1980
31. Lehman JF, Warren CG, Schom SM: Therapeutic heat and cold. Clin Orthop 99:207, 1974
32. Swezey RL: Essentials of physical management and rehabilitation in arthritis. Sem Arthritis Rheum 3:349, 1974
33. Swezey RL: Exercises with a beach ball for increasing range of joint motion. Arch Phys Med Rehabil 48:253, 1967
34. Brewer EJ Jr, Blattner RJ, Wing H: Treatment of rheumatoid arthritis in children. Pediatr Clin North Am 10:207, 1963
35. Melvin JL, Brannan KL, LeRoy EC: Comprehensive care for the patient with systemic sclerosis. Clin Rheum Prac 2:112, 1984
36. Oakes TW, Ward JR, Gray RM, et al: Family expectations and arthritis patient compliance to a hand resting splint regimen. Chronic Dis 20:757, 1970
37. Litt IF, Cluskey WP, Rosenberg A: Role of self-esteem and autonomy in determining medication compliance among adolescents with juvenile rheumatoid arthritis. Pediatrics 69:15, 1982
38. Arthritis Medical Information Series. Arthritis in Children. Arthritis Foundation, Atlanta, 1983
39. Sullivan DB, Ragsdale GG, Barnes L, et al: Juvenile Rheumatoid Arthritis: What it is and how we're treating it. University of Michigan Regents, 1986

40. When Your Student Has Childhood Arthritis: A Guide for Teachers. Arthritis Foundation, Atlanta
41. Whitehouse R, Shope, JT, Kulik C, et al: The JRA child at school: functional problems and the implementation of PL 94-142. Proceedings ARA/AHPA Annual Scientific Meetings. Arthritis Foundation, 1982
42. Whitehouse R, Shope JT, Graham-Tomasi R, et al: Educational needs of school personnel working with children with juvenile rheumatoid arthritis. Proceedings ARA/AHPA Annual Scientific Meetings, Arthritis Foundation, 1983
43. Donovan WE: Physical measures in the treatment of rheumatoid arthritis. p. 209. In Miller JJ, (ed): Juvenile Rheumatoid Arthritis. Littleton, Massachusetts, 1979
44. Colachis JG, Strohn BR: Cervical spine motion in normal women: Radiographic study of effect of cervical collars. Arch Phys Med Rehabil 54:161, 1973
45. Scott RD, Sarakhan AJ, Dalziel R: Total hip and total knee arthroplasty in juvenile rheumatoid arthritis. Clin Orthop 182:90, 1984
46. Ansell B: Rehabilitation in juvenile chronic arthritis. Rheumatol Tindall 18:74, 1979
47. Eyring EJ, Langert A, Bass JG: Synovectomy in juvenile rheumatoid arthritis. J Bone Joint Surg 53A:638, 1971
48. Granberry WM, Brewer EJ Jr: Results of synovectomy in children with rheumatoid arthritis. Clin Orthop 101:120, 1974
49. Granberry WM: Synovectomy in juvenile rheumatoid arthritis. Arthritis Rheum (suppl) 20:561, 1977
50. Ansell BM, Swann M: The management of chronic arthritis of children. J Bone Joint Surg 65B:536, 1983
51. Ranawat CS, Bryan WJ, Inglis AE: Total knee arthroplasty in juvenile arthritis. Arthritis Rheum 26:1140, 1983
52. Scott RD, Sledge CB: The surgery of juvenile rheumatoid arthritis. p. 1910. In Kelley WN, Harris ED, Ruddy S, Sledge CB (eds): Textbook of Rheumatology. Vol. II. WB Saunders, Philadelphia, 1981
53. Singsen BH, Isaacson AS, Bernstein BH, et al: Total hip replacement in children with arthritis. Arthritis Rheum 20:401, 1978
54. Arden GP, Ansell BM, Hunter MJ: Total hip replacement in juvenile chronic polyarthritis and ankylosing spondylitis. Clin Orthop 84:130, 1972
55. Sledge CB: Joint replacement in juvenile rheumatoid arthritis. Arthritis Rheum (suppl) 20:567, 1977
56. Herring JA: Destructive arthritis of the hip in juvenile rheumatoid arthritis. J Pediatr Orthop 4:259, 1984
57. Ansell BM: Rehabilitation. p. 201. In Arden GP, Ansell BM (eds): Surgical Management of Juvenile Chronic Polyarthritis. Grune & Stratton, Orlando, FL, 1978
58. Petty RE: Spondyloarthropathies. p. 283. In Cassidy JT (ed): Textbook of Pediatric Rheumatology. John Wiley & Sons, New York, 1982
59. Schaller JG: Ankylosing spondylitis of childhood onset. Arthritis Rheum (suppl) 20:398, 1977
60. Schaller JG, Omenn GS: The histocompatibility system and human disease. J Pediatr 88:913, 1976
61. Jacobs P: Ankylosing spondylitis in children and adolescents. Arch Dis Child 38:492, 1963
62. Blumberg R, Ragan C: Natural history of rheumatoid spondylitis. Medicine 35:1, 1956
63. Schaller JG, Bitnum S, Wedgwood RJ: Ankylosing spondylitis with childhood onset. J Pediatr 74:505, 1969

64. Macrae IF, Wright V: Measurement of back movement. Ann Rheum Dis 28:584, 1969
65. Frost M, Stuckey S, Smalley LA, Dorman G: Reliability of measuring trunk motion in centimeters. Phys Ther 62:1431, 1982
66. Bywaters EGL: Ankylosing spondylitis in childhood: Clin Rheum Dis. 2:387, 1976
67. Sullivan DB: Dermatomyositis. p. 407. In Cassidy, JT (ed): Textbook of Pediatric Rheumatology. John Wiley & Sons, New York, 1982
68. Pearson CM: Polymyositis. Annu Rev Med 17:63, 1969
69. Hanson V, Kornreich H: Systemic rheumatic disorders ("collagen disease") in childhood: Lupus erythematosis, anaphylactoid purpura, dermatomyositis, and scleroderma. Bull Rheum Dis 17:441, 1967
70. Sullivan DB, Cassidy JT, Petty RE, Burt A: Prognosis in childhood dermatomyositis. J Pediatr 80:555, 1972
71. Rose AL: Childhood polymyositis. Dis Child 127:518, 1974
72. Bitnum S, Daeschner CW, Travis LB, et al: Dermatomyositis. J Pediatr 64:101, 1964
73. Jacobs JC: Treatment of dermatomyositis. Arthritis Rheum 20:338, 1977
74. Cook CD, Rosen FS, Banker BQ: Dermatomyositis and focal scleroderma. Pediatr Clin North Am 10:979, 1963
75. Hill RH, Wood WS: Juvenile dermatomyositis. Can Med Assoc J 103:1152, 1970
76. Vanace PW: Chronic-state treatment of dermatomyositis. Arthritis Rheum (suppl) 20:342, 1977
77. Dabich L: Scleroderma. p. 433. In Cassidy JT (ed): Textbook of Pediatric Rheumatology. John Wiley & Sons, New York, 1982
78. Dabich L, Sullivan DB, Cassidy JT: Scleroderma in the child. J Pediatr 85:770, 1974
79. Hanson V: Systemic lupus erythematosis, dermatomyositis, scleroderma, and vasculitides in childhood. p. 1293. In Kelley WN, Harris ED, Ruddy S, Sledge CB: Textbook of Rheumatology, Vol. II. WB Saunders, Philadelphia, 1981
80. Cassidy JT, Sullivan DB, Dabich L, Petty RE: Scleroderma in children. Arthritis Rheum 20:351, 1977
81. Subcommittee for Scleroderma Criteria, American Rheumatism Association, Diagnostic and Therapeutic Criteria Committee: Preliminary criteria for the classification of systemic sclerosis (scleroderma). Bull Rheum Dis 31:1, 1981
82. Chazen EM, Cook CD, Cohen J: Focal scleroderma. J Pediatr 60:385, 1962
83. Medsger TA Jr, Masi AT, Rodnan GP, et al: Survival with systemic sclerosis (scleroderma). Ann Intern Med 75:369, 1971
84. Beng RL: Case report: Use of skin grafting to keep a scleroderma patient ambulant. Plas Reconstr Surg 63:732, 1979
85. Entin MA, Wilkinson RD: Scleroderma hand: A reappraisal. Orthop Clin North Am. 4:1031, 1973
86. Rudolph RI, Leyden JJ: Physiatrics for deforming linear scleroderma. Arch Dermatol 112:995, 1976

Appendix 1: Physical Therapy Protocol for Rheumatoid Arthritis

Linda K. Schroeder

I. Purpose
  A. Provide initial and continued assessment of
    1. Range of joint motion
    2. Strength
    3. Functional mobility
    4. Gait pattern
  B. Provide treatment and/or home program instruction to
    1. Relieve pain
    2. Improve joint motion
    3. Improve muscle strength
    4. Improve functional level
    5. Improve gait pattern
    6. Prevent deformity
    7. Maximize respiratory function

II. Assessment procedures
  A. History
    1. Previous physical therapy
    2. Previous home program and compliance
    3. Orthotic splints or shoes and compliance

    B. Foot assessment
- 1. Pain
- 2. Joint stability
- 3. Deformity

    C. Mobility assessment (note equipment used)
- 1. Bed mobility
- 2. Transfers
- 3. Functional ambulation
- 4. Gait

    D. Therapeutic programs done at home
- 1. Exercises
- 2. Modalities

    E. Range of motion
- 1. Note subluxed joints
- 2. Note influencing factors
  - a. Pain
  - b. Swelling
  - c. Crepitus
  - d. Time of test
  - e. Analgesics

    F. Strength
- 1. Manual muscle testing
  - a. Usually major muscle groups only
  - b. Note when pain or joint problems influence test
  - c. May test in non-standard positions when limited by pain or mobility restriction
- 2. Cybex (Lumex Inc., Ronkonkoma, NY) test
  - a. Quadricep and hamstring test at 30/sec. when objective documentation required
  - b. Should not be attempted with acutely inflamed joints
- 3. Hand strength assessment
  - a. Grip strength
    - (1) Adapted sphygmomanometer
    - (2) Manual resistance to grip
  - b. Formal muscle test

    G. Respiratory function
- 1. Respiratory rate and pattern
  - a. At rest
  - b. With exercise
- 2. Further evaluation if acute problems present

III. Treatment procedures

    A. Modalities: use prior to exercise or mobility to decrease pain and facilitate movement
- 1. Heat
  - a. Hydrocollator (Chattanooga Corp., Hixon, TN) packs

      b. Paraffin
      c. Moistaire cabinet, caution: increased cardiac stress
      d. Hydrotherapy, caution: increased cardiac stress with full body immersion
      e. Diathermy and ultrasound: contraindicated over joints
      f. Adaptations for home
  2. Cold
      a. Contraindicated with Raynaud's phenomenon
      b. Ice pack
      c. Ice massage
      d. Adaptations for home
  3. Heat-cold combination: contrast baths
  4. Massage
  5. Transcutaneous electrical nerve stimulation: high rate
B. Exercise
  1. Range of motion
      a. Types
          (1) Passive
          (2) Assistive
          (3) Active
          (4) Mechanical assist (eg, pulleys)
      b. Force: gentle passive force at end of range
      c. Preferred timing
          (1) When stiffness subsides
             (a) Later morning
             (b) After use of heat or ice
          (2) First thing in the morning if exercise diminishes stiffness
      d. Frequency
          (1) Daily minimum
          (2) Two to ten repetitions of exercises
          (3) Incorporate into entire day
      e. Pain
          (1) May increase with exercise
          (2) *Increased* pain should not persist more than 2 or 3 hours after exercise
  2. Strength
      a. Isometric
          (1) Minimal joint strain
          (2) Safe and convenient
          (3) Caution: increased cardiac stress
      b. Isotonics
          (1) Use only when pain or supporting structures are not a problem
          (2) Resistive exercises: use caution regarding joint forces
          (3) Goal directed to improve function, not to increase muscle bulk

3. Relaxation exercises
   a. Quick techniques involving imagery and breathing
   b. Jacobson's exercises
4. Breathing exercises
   a. When lung involvement present
   b. To promote relaxation
   c. Coordinate with exercise
5. Conditioning exercises
   a. Preliminary: marching, dancing, or other movement exercises while sitting
   b. Overall: swimming
   c. Advanced: stationary bicycle
6. Recreational exercise
   a. Consider specific joints involved and disease process
   b. Consider cardiovascular and circulatory impairments
   c. Consider stress and impact of activity
   d. Consider energy requirements and patterns involved in specific recreational exercise
   e. Instruct in analysis of specific recreational exercise in relationship to patient's condition
   f. Reinforce principles of activity pacing

C. Posture and mobility
   1. Recommend equipment and orthoses to achieve mobility goals
   2. Posture and positioning instruction
   3. Body mechanics instruction
   4. Bed mobility training
   5. Transfer training
   6. Functional mobility training
   7. Shoe and foot orthosis recommendations
   8. Gait training

D. Follow-up
   1. Written home program provided
   2. Equipment needs addressed
   3. Family instruction provided as needed
   4. Home physical therapy arranged when indicated
   5. Out-patient physical therapy when indicated

Appendix 2: Physical Therapy Protocol for Ankylosing Spondylitis

Linda K. Schroeder

I. Goals
  A. To provide initial and continued assessment of
    1. Range of joint motion
    2. Posture
    3. Chestwall mobility
    4. Muscle strength
    5. Gait pattern
    6. Functional level
  B. To maximize available joint motion and flexibility
  C. To improve strength
  D. To maximize posture and alignment
  E. To facilitate maximum level of function
  F. To improve ambulation and mobility
  G. To decrease pain
  H. To improve chest expansion

II. Evaluation
  A. Posture (observe in standing)
    1. Cervical
    2. Thoracic
    3. Lumbar

        4. Lateral symmetry
        5. Height
B. Spine mobility
        1. Cervical flexion
           a. Measure distance: chin to sternal notch
           b. Record in centimeters
        2. Cervical extension
           a. Measure distance: occipital protuberance to C7
           b. Record in centimeters
        3. Cervical rotation
           a. Normal is 80°
           b. Approximate range: full, three-quarter, one-half, one-quarter
           c. Measure left and right
        4. Cervical lateral flexion
           a. Measure distance: tragus to posterior tip of acromion
           b. Record in centimeters
           c. Measure left and right
        5. Trunk rotation
           a. Evaluate in sitting
           b. Normal is 40°
           c. Approximate range: full, three-quarter, one-half, one-quarter
        6. Trunk lateral flexion
           a. Evaluate standing, heels 7 inches apart
           b. Measure distance: middle finger to knee joint line
           c. Record distance in centimeters above or below knee joint
        7. Forward flexion
           a. Evaluate standing, heels 7 inches apart, knees straight
           b. Measure distance: middle finger to floor
           c. Record in centimeters
        8. Schober test
           a. With patient standing erect
              (1) Mark lumbosacral junction
              (2) Mark location 10 cm above junction
           b. With patient bent forward (spine fully flexed) measure distance between two marks
           c. Record distance in centimeters
           d. Normal is greater than 15 cm
        9. Occiput to wall
           a. Evaluate with patient standing, heels against wall, chin horizontal
           b. Patient attempts to touch wall with occiput
           c. Measure distance from occiput to wall
           d. Record in centimeters
           e. Normal is 0 cm
       10. Chest expansion

        a. Measure chest circumference at level of xiphoid process during full inspiration and full expiration

        b. Record difference between full inspiration and full expiration in centimeters

        c. Normal is 5 cm

C. Peripheral joint range of motion/muscle tightness
1. Shoulders
2. Hips: check for hip flexor tightness
3. Other joints

D. Strength
1. Back extensors
2. Scapular adductors
3. Hip extensors

E. Gait

F. Functional mobility

III. Treatment

  A. Posture
1. Sitting/standing
   a. Emphasize erect posture
   b. Minimize trunk and neck flexion postures
      (1) Leaning over desk
      (2) Gardening
   c. Proper seating to encourage erect posture
   d. Encourage breaks from flexed postures
      (1) Axial extension
      (2) Scapular retraction
      (3) Trunk extension
      (4) Hip extension
2. Rest/sleep
   a. Firm support
   b. Minimize neck and head support when supine
   c. Encourage extension postures
   d. Encourage breaks from flexed postures
      (1) 15-minute supine or prone rest breaks
      (2) 15 minutes supine or prone before and after sleep (if unable to sleep supine)

  B. Exercise
1. Range of motion/flexibility
   a. Trunk/neck
      (1) Extension (active and passive)
      (2) Cervical axial extension
      (3) Rotation
      (4) Lateral flexion
   b. Extremities
      (1) Shoulders
      (2) Hips
      (3) Other

      2. Strengthening
        a. Scapular adduction
        b. Back extension
        c. Hip extension
        d. Other
      3. Respiratory
        a. Lateral costal expansion
        b. Upper chest expansion
        c. Breathing retraining
      4. Relaxation training
      5. Recreational exercise
        a. Encourage
        b. Appropriate to severity and course of disease
        c. Select activities that reinforce treatment goals for posture, strength, and flexibility
        d. Balance unilateral activities (archery, golf) with exercises to other side
        e. Avoid hard physical contact
        f. Avoid activities with repetitive impact loading of joints (jogging, handball, trampoline)
      6. Exercise precautions
        a. Avoid trunk flexion exercise
        b. During periods of joint swelling and inflammation limit exercise to range of motion
        c. Spine flexibility exercises may need to be changed as disease progresses (no longer safe)
        d. Sudden sharp pain may indicate fracture of ankylosed segment: prompt physician assessment
C. Modalities
      1. Ice
      2. Superficial heat
        a. Local: hot packs
        b. General: hydrotherapy
      3. Diathermy (administered by physical therapists)
        a. Use over muscle spasm only
        b. Avoid use over enthesopathic inflammation
      4. Massage
      5. High rate transcutaneous electrical nerve stimulation
D. Mobility and gait
      1. Gait training
      2. Transfer training
      3. Wheelchair mobility training
      4. Bed mobility training
E. Home program instruction
      1. Self evaluation
        a. Height
        b. Chest expansion
      2. Treatment as noted above

Appendix 3: Physical Therapy Protocol for Polymyositis/ Dermatomyositis

Linda K. Schroeder

The physical therapy treatment of polymyositis/dermatomyositis is dependent on the level of disease activity, muscle inflammation, and respiratory impairment. Communication with the patient's rheumatologist is important to determine when the patient's medical condition has improved sufficiently to progress treatment. Physical therapists should continue to monitor creatine kinase (CK) blood levels, strength, respiration, and endurance.

I. Acute phase
   A. Clinical presentation
      1. CK levels may be elevated, indicating muscle inflammation (normal = 0–225)
      2. Proximal muscles weaker than distal muscles
      3. Muscle pain
   B. Activity level
      1. Strict bed rest
      2. Minimal active movement
   C. Goals
      1. Document strength

   2. Optimal respiratory function
   3. Increase range of motion, prevent contractures
   4. Decrease pain
   5. Improve relaxation
   D. Treatment location
   1. Bedside
   2. Cybex (Lumex Inc., Ronkonkoma, NY) strength assessment in physical therapy department
   E. Treatment
   1. Serial strength assessment
       a. Manual muscle testing
           (1) Proximal and distal groups
           (2) Limit number of muscles tested to avoid fatigue
       b. Cybex strength assessment
           (1) Quadriceps and hamstrings
           (2) Triceps and biceps
           (3) Speed: 30°/sec
   2. Respiratory assessment and treatment of impairment
   3. Range of motion assessment and treatment
       a. *Passive range* of motion of all extremities and trunk
       b. *Avoid* active and active assistive exercise
       c. Gentle joint mobilization and stretching
   4. Pain treatments
       a. Transcutaneous electrical nerve stimulation (TENS) may be used in conjunction with shoulder stretch
       b. TENS may be used to decrease back pain
       c. Massage to relax muscle spasm
   5. Relaxation instruction
       a. Avoid the contraction phase of Jacobson's technique
       b. Breathing techniques
       c. Imagery

II. Recovering phase
   A. Clinical presentation
   1. CK level decreasing if previously elevated
   2. Strength improving
   3. Muscle pain decreasing
   B. Activity level
   1. No longer on strict bed rest
   2. Limited sitting and mobility at bedside
   C. Additional goals
   1. Functional assessment
   2. Equipment recommendations
   3. Independence in home program
   4. Follow-up arranged
   D. Treatment location

        1. Bedside

        2. Nursing unit

   E. Treatment

        1. Functional training

            a. Minimize to avoid fatigue

            b. Family instruction in any needed assistance

        2. Equipment needs assessed and identified

        3. Range of motion home program

            a. Begin active exercise

            b. 1 to 3 repetitions only

        4. Back pain home program

            a. Abdominal isometrics: 1 to 3 repetitions only

            b. Posture and body mechanics instruction

            c. Corset, but must not impair respiratory function

            d. TENS

        5. Follow-up arranged

III. Rehabilitation phase

   A. Clinical presentation

        1. Return of CK to normal if previously elevated

        2. Maintenance of normal CK during steroid taper

        3. Strength continues increasing: documented by Cybex

        4. Disease inactive

   B. Acitivity level: gradually increased

   C. Additional goals

        1. Increase strength

        2. Maximize function

   D. Treatment location

        1. Out-patient physical therapy

        2. Home program

   E. Treatment

        1. Strengthening

        2. Advanced mobility training

Index

Page numbers followed by *f* denote figures; those followed by *t* denote tables.

PHYSICAL THERAPY
MANAGEMENT
of ARTHRITIS

CLINICS IN PHYSICAL THERAPY
VOLUME 16